It's Not Just About The Food!

How To Get Off the Diet Rollercoaster and Create the Life and Body You Want

By Mark Shepard, NLPT

Mark Shepard, NLPT—Master Practitioner & Trainer of NLP, Hypnosis & Time Line Therapy™:
Rapid Results for Individual and Organizational Empowerment & Transformation
ItsNotJustAboutTheFood.com Copyright 2003, 2004, 2005, 2013, 2014 by Mark Shepard All Rights Reserved

The Materials In This Program:

- **It's Not Just About The Food!** How to Get off the Diet Roller Coaster and Create The Body and Life You Love With NLP & Hypnosis. Workbook $47.00

- **It's Not Just About The Food!** CD $47.00

- **Thirsty For the Sky**: Songs of Empowerment and Healing. Mark's original songs to be used for support and reinforcement CD $20

- **Eyes on the Horizon**: More songs of empowerment and healing. CD $20.

- **Weight Loss Hypnosis induction**. to be used for continual reinforcement. CD $47.00

- **NLP Tools For Transformation: Swish Patterns, Anchoring, Submodality Shifts**. Use this Cd whenever you need to fine tune your brain. $47.00

- **Time Line Therapy™ Clearing Negative Emotions, Limiting Decisions and Anxiety** CD. Use this CD to guide you in clearing your negative emotions, limiting decisions, Anxiety and more. $47.00

Total cost if purchased separately $275.00 Your price? $99.99

According to US estimates from The National Institute of Mental Health, between 5 per cent and 10 per cent of girls and women (i.e. 5-10 million people) and 1 million boys and men suffer from eating disorders, including anorexia, bulimia, binge eating disorder, or other associated dietary conditions. Estimates suggest that as many as 15 percent of young women adopt unhealthy attitudes and behaviors about food.

In addition:

- An estimated 10 per cent of female college students suffer from a clinical or sub-clinical (borderline) eating disorder, of which over half suffer from bulimia nervosa.
- An estimated 1 in 100 American women binges and purges to lose weight.
- Approximately 5 per cent of women and 1 percent of men have anorexia nervosa, bulimia nervosa, or binge eating disorder.
- 15 per cent of young women have significantly disordered eating attitudes and behavior.
- It is estimated that 200,000 to 300,000 Canadian women aged 13 to 40 have anorexia nervosa and twice as many have bulimia.
- Studies suggest that 5 to 10 percent of people with anorexia or bulimia are males.
- An estimated 1 in 3 of all dieters develop compulsive dieting attitudes and behaviors. Of these, one quarter will develop full or partial eating disorders.
- In the UK, nearly 2 in every 100 secondary school girls suffer from anorexia nervosa, bulimia nervosa or binge eating disorder.
- Due to the incidence of co-occurring medical conditions, it is almost impossible to specify the morbidity rates for eating disorders like anorexia, bulimia or binge eating. However, general estimates suggest that as many as 10-15 per cent of eating disorders are fatal for those affected.
- Each day Americans spend an average of $109 million on dieting and diet related products.

> Between 5-10 million girls and women and 1 million boys and men in the US suffer from eating disorders, including anorexia, bulimia, binge eating disorder, or other associated dietary conditions.

Source http://www.annecollins.com/eating-disorders/statistics.htm

Mark Shepard, NLPT—Master Practitioner & Trainer of NLP, Hypnosis & Time Line Therapy™:
Rapid Results for Individual and Organizational Empowerment & Transformation
ItsNotJustAboutTheFood.com Copyright 2003, 2004, 2005, 2013, 2014 by Mark Shepard All Rights Reserved

Table of Contents:

Mark Shepard, NLPT—Master Practitioner & Trainer of NLP, Hypnosis & Time Line Therapy™:
Rapid Results for Individual and Organizational Empowerment & Transformation
ItsNotJustAboutTheFood.com Copyright 2003, 2004, 2005, 2013, 2014 by Mark Shepard All Rights Reserved

Chapter One

It's Not Just About The Food

Mark Shepard, NLPT—Master Practitioner & Trainer of NLP, Hypnosis & Time Line Therapy™:
Rapid Results for Individual and Organizational Empowerment & Transformation
ItsNotJustAboutTheFood.com Copyright 2003, 2004, 2005, 2013, 2014 by Mark Shepard All Rights Reserved

It's Not Just About The Food

Think about it! In our country today, despite the 3 gazillion new diets and the eruption of millions of exercise studios & gyms we are a nation of overweight people and we just seem to keep gaining weight.

Since 2003, most of the clients I've worked with in my private practice have been on all the diets. Atkins. Pritikin. The Zone. The Scarsdale Diet. The Grapefruit Diet. You name it. They've tried it...

They should be called, "The Yo-Yo Diet" or "The Roller Coaster Diet" or "The Starve Yourself Until You Can't Stand It and Then Binge" Diet!

They have tried working out. But after a few days of forcing themselves to go to the gym they either just lose interest or hurt themselves so they have to stop...

> Between 5-10 million girls and women and 1 million boys and men in the US suffer from eating disorders, including anorexia, bulimia, binge eating disorder, or other associated dietary conditions.

They've tried the shakes. They've tried the pills and powders.

Many have even considered or had dangerous surgical procedures....

Nothing seems to help. Theoretically if you take in fewer calories that you use on a daily basis, you "should" lose weight, right?

Mark Shepard, NLPT—Master Practitioner & Trainer of NLP, Hypnosis & Time Line Therapy™:
Rapid Results for Individual and Organizational Empowerment & Transformation
ItsNotJustAboutTheFood.com Copyright 2003, 2004, 2005, 2013, 2014 by Mark Shepard All Rights Reserved

So all you have to do, the experts say, is eat less and exercise more...

If it's so simple why aren't we all doing it?

Here are a few reasons:

1. **Your body is an amazing survival mechanism.** When you go on a reduced calorie diet, it signals to your body that there is a potential lack, famine, risk of starvation, DANGER.

   So it gets really efficient. It readjusts the "Set Point" of your metabolism to burn the body's stored energy reserves very frugally.

   "Make it last!," your body hears. "We don't know when the next meal is coming from..."

An estimated 1 in 3 of all dieters develop compulsive dieting attitudes and behaviors.

Of these, one quarter will develop full or partial eating disorders.

Throughout the course of our evolution people who had the ability to survive on very little were the ones who lived to pass on their genes to the next generation.

Then comes the abundance of the last 50-100 years and what once helped us survive now begins to threaten the very lives it's designed to protect.

"Fine", you say, "if there's ever a famine in our country I'll be the one to survive and all you skinny people will finally stop annoying me..."

But the reality is that we live amidst unprecedented abundance of food...particularly cheap grain based

Mark Shepard, NLPT—Master Practitioner & Trainer of NLP, Hypnosis & Time Line Therapy™:
Rapid Results for Individual and Organizational Empowerment & Transformation
ItsNotJustAboutTheFood.com Copyright 2003, 2004, 2005, 2013, 2014 by Mark Shepard All Rights Reserved

carbs and multiple forms of sugar. Most of which, ironically is not just very low in nutritional value, it's downright poisonous to our bodies and often actually creates and exacerbates weight retention.

One of the things we'll do in this program is to change your set point and boost your resting metabolism so that you can burn off the stored energy we call "fat" even while you are sitting still.

In order to do this we will use the sophisticated (yet easy to learn) leading edge techniques of NLP, Hypnosis, Time Line Therapy™ and EFT. You will also learn how to re-inforce this internal change on a daily basis.

> Each day Americans spend an average of $109 million on dieting and diet related products.

2. **Sedentary Lifestyles:** We sit in front of computers and we sit in meetings and we sit in cars then we come home and sit in front of the TV...a lot.

A body at rest tends to stay at rest.

To begin the shift to being the body in motion that tends to stay in motion, we will use hypnosis to install a literal "thirst for movement" so that whether you are regularly going to the gym or not, you will begin to add extra movement into your life.

Remember when you were a kid and always wanted to play? What happened to that? When did exercise become work? What if you started thinking about moving your body as "recess" or "playtime" and eagerly looked forward to doing it every day?

Mark Shepard, NLPT—Master Practitioner & Trainer of NLP, Hypnosis & Time Line Therapy™:
Rapid Results for Individual and Organizational Empowerment & Transformation
ItsNotJustAboutTheFood.com Copyright 2003, 2004, 2005, 2013, 2014 by Mark Shepard All Rights Reserved

3. **Old negative and limiting beliefs about ourselves**, unresolved childhood trauma, and perceptual filters that cause us to give up too soon and sabotage what progress we make. A lot of times when working with my private clients the changes we make in these "old programs" create massive positive results in every area of their lives.

   In this program you'll make a significant dent in clearing these old programs. I will teach you simple and powerful techniques that will enable you to recognize when a "limiting decision" is at work and how to literally erase it and re-program yourself.

4. **Stress and Anxiety:** How many of us are trying to cram too much stuff into each day to the extent that we are feeling like a gerbil running on an endless wheel of work, responsibilities, deadlines, and pressure?

   We will explore how to shift the internal beliefs that keep you from saying "no". You will also learn how to relax yourself and carry a sense of calm and well being through your day.

5. **Problem foods:** What's a problem food for you? For me it was homemade chocolate chip cookies. My grandmother made them for me...and put them in the freezer for when I visited her. So I would eat them one after another. I was a chain cookie eater...I associated the cookies with LOVE!...

   Now, I can still fondly remember my grandmother but I just don't find chocolate chip cookies appealing...We will use some powerful techniques from Neuro Linguistic Programming (NLP) to literally re-program your food likes and dislikes.

6. **Poor Nutrition:** You may have heard in numerous places about the lack of proper nutrients in our soils. Even or-

Mark Shepard, NLPT—Master Practitioner & Trainer of NLP, Hypnosis & Time Line Therapy™:
Rapid Results for Individual and Organizational Empowerment & Transformation
ItsNotJustAboutTheFood.com

9

ganic produce does not have all the nutrients we need for the optimal functioning of our cells.

We will be exploring how to specific foods, herbal supplements and vitamins can assist you to nourish your cells and boost your metabolism pleasurably (and affordably).

7. **Goal setting and keeping track of our positive results**. Most people set unrealistic goals or use an ineffective goal setting process.

Then they forget to notice the positive changes in their lives and instead focus on the setbacks.

Unfortunately our neurology is designed to deliver what we focus on. So re-training ourselves to focus on even the small positive changes rather than the reverse is crucial for any long term success whether it's weight loss, creating better careers, or relationships for ourselves. We will be using leading edge techniques from NLP & Time Line Therapy™ in this segment to literally program our future.

8. **Helpless, hopeless, victim thinking.** One of the main tasks of this program (as well as with my work with clients in other areas) is to help you get to the place where _you are in charge of your life_.

This includes your thoughts. If we think we can't succeed we are already half beaten. I will do my best to help you shake yourself out of this. I will sing to you. I will nudge you. I will challenge you. This piece is crucial.

So, imagine the roller coaster car slowing down and coming to a halt...

Push away the restraining bar...

Climb out onto solid ground and begin to walk with me through a

Mark Shepard, NLPT—Master Practitioner & Trainer of NLP, Hypnosis & Time Line Therapy™:
Rapid Results for Individual and Organizational Empowerment & Transformation

process of self transformation that has positive implications for every area of your life!

As we proceed down the path to creating a slim, fit, vibrant, healthy body that will be yours for your full lifetime, imagine feeling light on your feet, your clothes, loose and comfortable, breathing deep full breaths and just feeling calm and relaxed...

But wait!

Before your unconscious mind gets so enthusiastic about making those changes you want inside that it decides to just *go ahead and make those changes* now...

Who the heck am I to be your coach through this process? Why should you *pay attention* to what I have to say?

Thanks for asking! I appreciate your candor.

Turn the page and I'll do my best to answer...

Chapter Two
Meet Your Coach:
Mark Shepard, NLPT

If you are asking yourself, "Who the heck is Mark Shepard and why should I listen to him?", then read this:

I came to NLP, Hypnosis and Time Line Therapy™ by a lifelong journey of pain, frustration, depression, anxiety, limiting beliefs and self-defeating behaviors.

Although I was never seriously overweight until I hit my late 40's, I had numerous food allergies, I was totally addicted to sweets and simple carbs I had serious digestive issues, bloating, gas, constipation and frequent abdominal pain. I tried a lot of different diets to try to correct the problem but never seemed to make progress.

Ever feel like you have no energy? Like you are dragging heavy chains around with you wherever you go? I know that feeling!

I could barely make it through the day without a nap.

Then, I would sleep 9 or 10 hours. Having so little energy made me depressed because I knew that without a high energy level I would never achieve my dream of making it in the music business.

Being depressed robbed me of even more energy so I would turn to Chocolate Chip Cookies or Starbucks Java Chip Ice Cream for soothing.

Does this kind of vicious cycle sound or feel familiar to you? Where I was then probably didn't look much different than where you are now.

The main source of my pain was my seeming inability to get my songs out into the world.

I couldn't' handle criticism or rejection.

And I interpreted EVERYTHING as criticism and rejection. The very thought of picking up the phone and calling ANYONE much less a record company or booking agent sent me deep into panic and fear, which would cause me to "self-medicate" with cookies and ice cream.

In relationships, I just could not speak my truth, I held on to negative emotions like anger and resentment. At the same time I was dependent and needy... I couldn't speak up for my needs or express my truth. So I held it all in and, yup you guessed it, self soothed with cookies and ice cream.

In almost every area of my life I was the epitome of a victim.

Mark Shepard, NLPT—Master Practitioner & Trainer of NLP, Hypnosis & Time Line Therapy™:
Rapid Results for Individual and Organizational Empowerment & Transformation
ItsNotJustAboutTheFood.com Copyright 2003, 2004, 2005, 2013, 2014 by Mark Shepard All Rights Reserved

Financially I was a ruin. I'd bought four houses for nothing down at the top of the 1980's real estate bubble. Shortly after buying them the bubble burst and I ended up owing more on them than they were worth.

Eventually I lost everything, my home, my marriage...

In other words I was a mess, maybe even more of a mess than you think you are...

In the late 1980's I tried psychotherapy with little progress. Talking about my problems just seemed to make them worse and I had no health insurance so I basically couldn't afford to spend week after week just talking.

I needed results.

Then I stumbled onto a book by a former NASA physicist named Barbara Brennan called "Hands of Light".

Since she was a physicist she seemed to bring a lot of credibility to this wild notion that there is something called "healing energy."

I eventually found one of her students, Mearah Marqua to work with. I began studying energy healing with her one weekend a month. Slowly things began to change. And I continued to study with other healers (one of whom, Suzanne Scott, used a pendulum to test me for food allergies).

Within a week or two of following Suzanne's recommendations to cut out grains, junk foods like cookies and even fruit (which I thought was good for me), I had about 50% more energy).

I also read everything I could get my hands on about healing, personal empowerment, success, etc.

Eventually, I stumbled on the books of Anthony Robbins who introduced me to NLP.

Still it was many years before I actually began to pursue that path. When I finally did I was amazed at the rapidity with which I was able to make positive changes.

After discovering the power of NLP to make rapid, dramatic changes in the way I perceived the world, I was on a tear to learn absolutely everything I could about this subject. So I read books, I bought audio programs and I eventually got the opportunity to study intensively in person with world renowned Master Trainer of NLP, & Hypnosis, Tad James. Tad James is also the creator of Time Line Therapy ™.

To be honest with you it would take me a whole book to tell you this story fully and I know you aren't here to learn about <u>me</u> so much as you are to **get off the Diet Rollercoaster and get your life and body in order.**

The point I want to make though is that the tools I offer here <u>work</u>! **If you work them** of course.

The very fact that I have an uneaten package of chocolate chip cookies in my cabinet that someone gave to me several months ago should tell you something.

In the past, if there were <u>any</u> chocolate chip cookies in the house, I would find them and I would eat them one after another until they were gone...Then I would actually wonder where they went! That's just one tiny example of the changes I've manifested in my life using these cutting edge tools for transformation.

So why should you listen to me?

Only because the information in this book and CD series <u>works</u>. It works spectacularly and not just for weight loss and fitness... The principles here will work for you in any area of your life where you desire change.

Are you ready to learn about "the tools of transformation" in our tool kit so you can change your life now?

Then turn the page!

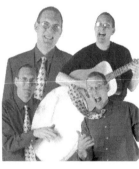

About Mark Shepard:

Your instructor: Mark Shepard, CHt, PhD(c), NLPT is a master practitioner and trainer of Hypnosis, NLP & Time Line Therapy™. His training style puts people immediately at ease and utilizes leading edge presentation techniques to "layer in" information in a way that is easily and effortlessly integrated on the conscious and unconscious level. He also incorporates storytelling and original songs into his teaching methods. In other words, **Mark makes learning easy and fun** which increases retention and utilization of the material. In addition to his training, consulting and speaking work, **Shepard maintains a private practice in Albany, NY** where he assists his clients achieve their financial, health and relationship goals.

Chapter Three
The Turbo Tools
of Transformation

Mark Shepard, NLPT—Master Practitioner & Trainer of NLP, Hypnosis & Time Line Therapy™:
Rapid Results for Individual and Organizational Empowerment & Transformation

Neuro Linguistic Programming
(a.k.a. NLP)
What the heck is it and why should you care?

NLP is to personal transformation what Pilates is to fitness, what BOSE is to stereo systems, what the laser beam is to lighting.

It has been called "the study of excellence." (Tad James, PhD)

It has been said that "NLP is an attitude and a methodology that leaves behind a trail of techniques" (Richard Bandler, PhD, co-founder of NLP)

In my opinion, NLP is a model of internal and external communication that enables rapid and profound change. NLP is about consistently achieving our desired outcomes in all areas of our lives.

Some approaches focus on "why" we do something. NLP focuses on "how" we run our brains in order to do a certain behavior.

NLP is currently being used by many world class athletes, an increasing number of our world leaders and top business and arts professionals. I use NLP with my weight loss clients to assist them in literally "re-programming" habitual, self defeating behaviors, even changing what foods they like or dislike as well as how they respond to certain trigger situations.

"Yeah, yeah, yeah, but what is it really?"

In a nutshell, **NLP is about *how you run your brain*.**

Why should you care? Because it *works*. Once you learn how you create certain behaviors in your life you can also change them and create something different.

You do want to create something different don't you? That's why you're here right? There is literally nothing more effective on the planet. I know because I've searched.

I know beyond a shadow of a doubt that **everything that does work, works because of these principles regardless of what it's is called.**

Mark Shepard, NLPT—Master Practitioner & Trainer of NLP, Hypnosis & Time Line Therapy™:
Rapid Results for Individual and Organizational Empowerment & Transformation
ItsNotJustAboutTheFood.com Copyright 2003, 2004, 2005, 2013, 2014 by Mark Shepard All Rights Reserved

Hypnosis

is a useful state of heightened awareness enabling permanent, positive change, and activating our natural healing abilities.

It has been approved by the American Medical Association since 1958.

Hypnosis has tremendous implications for improving communication with the unconscious mind—where all change takes place.

Through hypnosis many weight loss clients find themselves easily able to stop behaviors that were previously compulsive and out of control.

We will be dispelling some of the myths about hypnosis (trust me, you will not be quacking like a duck at any point during this program unless you want to!) and exploring some of the amazing abilities of your unconscious mind.

We will also use Hypnosis to literally reprogram your "set point", adjust your metabolism and give your body permission to change into a fat burning and energy "wasting" vehicle.

Time Line Therapy™

is a leading edge transformation modality used worldwide for releasing traumatic emotions such as anger, grief and fear as well as limiting decisions, anxiety and phobias.

It has tremendous applications in clearing out the underlying causes of using food to self medicate or of failing to maintain a healthy fitness routine.

We also use it for literally "programming" future goals.

In some ways, Timeline is the perfect combination of NLP and Hypnosis. It's simplicity is misleading because it's effectiveness is often astonishing. In my opinion the discovery of the Time Line Therapy™ techniques will someday be considered one of the greatest discoveries of all time.

You will get to experience this for yourself.

EFT—Emotional Freedom Technique
(a.k.a. Meridian Tapping)

EFT, short for Emotional Freedom Technique or "Tapping" is a tool that works on a lot of different levels.

It is one of my favorite tools to use "in the moment" when "stuff is up" and you are face to face with a challenging emotional trigger situation.

What I like particularly about it is that you don't have to pretend to have a positive attitude! You can tap on the worst, negative, nasty stuff in your life and almost instantly feel actual, measurable relief.

There are a number of different levels and approaches to tapping that I've developed in my own life and working with clients over the years. I'll share them all with you in this program.

Mark Shepard, NLPT—Master Practitioner & Trainer of NLP, Hypnosis & Time Line Therapy™:
Rapid Results for Individual and Organizational Empowerment & Transformation
ItsNotJustAboutTheFood.com Copyright 2003, 2004, 2005, 2013, 2014 by Mark Shepard All Rights Reserved

NLP Communication Model

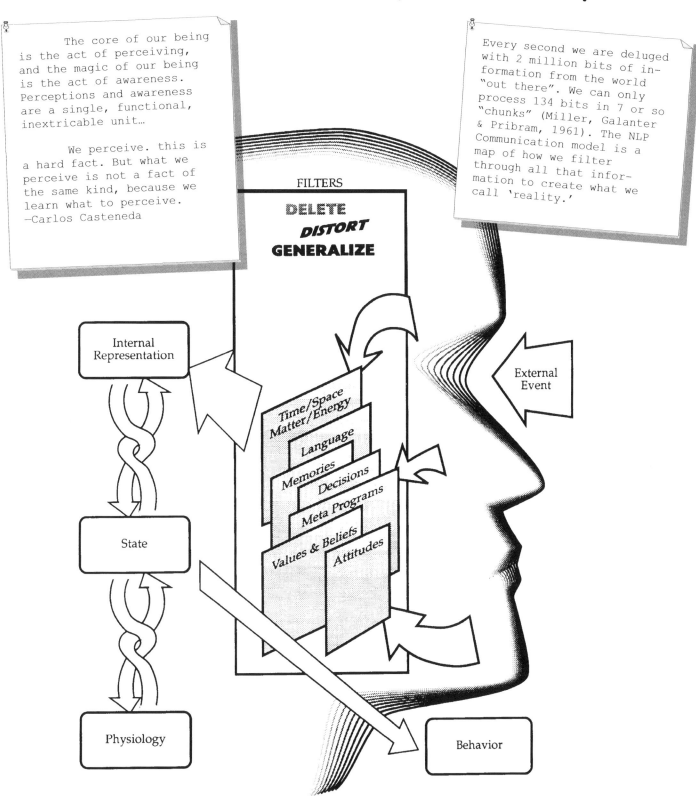

Typoglycemia

I cdnuolt blveiee taht I cluod aulaclty uesdnatnrd waht I was rdanieg. The phaonmneal pweor of the hmuan mnid. Aoccdrnig to a rscheearch at Cmabrigde Uinervtisy, it deosn't mttaer in-waht oredr the ltteers in a wrod are, the olny iprmoatnt tihng is taht the frist and lsat ltteer be in the rghit pclae. The rset can be a taotl mses and you can sitll raed it wouthit a porbelm. Tihs is bcuseae the huamn mnid deos not raed ervey lteter by istlef, but the wrod as a wlohe. Amzanig huh? yaeh and I awlyas thought slpeling was ipmorantt.

This is a good example of the phenomenal power of your mind to take the very hint of something and internally adjust it and create meaning.

This is the same process that happens when you see your spouse frown and "interpret" it to mean he or she is angry at you. You may be right but he or she may not even be thinking about you.

In working with clients who have a poor self image, I find they do this a lot. they take a tiny bit of information from other people, a whisper or a bit of sub-tle body language and build a negative experience from it.

We can also do the reverse. We can take a bit of information and conclude that other people are finding us likeable and attractive. Later on we'll learn how to do this and program the new way of interpreting the world into our neurology.

Chapter Four
"Getting to Cause:"
How To Stop
Being A Victim

Mark Shepard, NLPT—Master Practitioner & Trainer of NLP, Hypnosis & Time Line Therapy™:
Rapid Results for Individual and Organizational Empowerment & Transformation
ItsNotJustAboutTheFood.com Copyright 2003, 2004, 2005, 2013, 2014 by Mark Shepard All Rights Reserved

Taking Back Your Life,
"Getting To Cause"

So many of us go through our lives feeling trapped, helpless, hopeless and victimized . Little by little we give up on the dreams that used to seem so possible as kids. It seems as if our "default" program is to feel victimized by what happens to us. The media supports this notion. Every day we hear on the news about this "victim" or that "victim".

So many of us walk around with feelings of resentment and frustration that life isn't fair or that we didn't get what we wanted in life.

If we are in an unsatisfying relationship it's "just the way it is" or it's the other person's fault. If we aren't making enough money, well, mom and dad always said "money doesn't grow on trees."

Rich people are mean and selfish anyway, so why bother to try?

If we're overweight well it's our genes.

If we hate our job, well, you've got to eat right?

Doesn't <u>everybody</u> hate their job?

There <u>is</u> another approach.

And that is to begin to play with the idea that **we are the creators of our lives**.

For some this may be radical. In this belief system, if we experience an external event, **on some level we chose it.**

If we aren't making enough money there's a message we aren't listening to or there's a piece of us

---

It's Everyone's Fault but Mine.

"We have become a society of victims…

In Cleveland Ohio, a man sued M&M/Mars and a local candy dealer for $500,000.00 to cover hospitalization and surgery bills. He bit through his lip when he chomped down on an M&M peanut that did not have a peanut in it

In Boston, MA,. a would-be lifeguard, who is totally deaf, sued the YMCA for $20 million for prejudicially and insensitively requiring its lifeguards to be able to hear noises and distress signals.

In Raymondville, Texas, a man sued a dog owner for $25,000 after tripping over the dog in the man's kitchen, claiming the man neglected to warn him of the dog's propensity of lying in certain areas….

Few people will turn to themselves to take responsibility for their results until they have exhausted all opportunities to blame someone else"

From "Shut Up, Stop Whining & Get A Life by Larry Winget, John Wiley & Sons, 2004, pp13-14

Mark Shepard, NLPT—Master Practitioner & Trainer of NLP, Hypnosis & Time Line Therapy™:
Rapid Results for Individual and Organizational Empowerment & Transformation
ItsNotJustAboutTheFood.com Copyright 2003, 2004, 2005, 2013, 2014 by Mark Shepard All Rights Reserved

that resists success… If our significant other leaves us it's because on some level we needed to learn something or grow in some way. And the more we can appreciate this opportunity to learn the better.

By the way none of this is any more "True" than believing we are victims.

What it does do is give us a tremendous amount of power:
The power to choose how to respond to the events in our lives.

If **we** are the ones creating everything in our lives, then **we** can begin to create what we want rather than what we don't want.

Perception is Projection.
Whatever we are perceiving in our lives actually originated from within us. It is our interpretation of the world. It's as if there is nothing or nobody out there until we aim our internal movie projector outwards and switch on the light.

And every event, every person is simply a reflection of ourselves. If it's someone we admire, that's the brilliant or beautiful side of us. If It is someone we don't like or find annoying or unattractive, that's the part of ourselves that is either like that or fears being like that…

The point is not that any of it is "true".

The point is when we operate from this philosophy we are at cause, rather than effect. **We** are creating it. **It** is no longer "happening" to us. And by the way, the very fact that you are reading this means on some level you created it at this moment in your life to learn whatever… you…. need…to….learn ….**now.**

So let's roll up our sleeves and begin the process of…

Mark Shepard, NLPT—Master Practitioner & Trainer of NLP, Hypnosis & Time Line Therapy™:
Rapid Results for Individual and Organizational Empowerment & Transformation
ItsNotJustAboutTheFood.com Copyright 2003, 2004, 2005, 2013, 2014 by Mark Shepard All Rights Reserved

Getting To Cause...
Cause > Effect

Are you at cause in your life? Or are you a victim of this or that, or something else?

One of the most empowering ideas I've ever experienced is the notion that we are the creators of our lives. Whatever it is you are experiencing now has been created by you, by your thoughts, decisions, beliefs, focus, interpretations etc.

Even if you could prove to a jury of your peers that something was **done <u>to</u>** you, from this new point of view, **you still created it.** The point is no matter what happens in your life, when you "get to cause" and take "Response-Ability" for your outcomes, **you shift into a position of power.** You are no longer a victim and you never were one in the first place.

—**Mark Shepard**

"We may have been taught, and therefore have believed that we live at the mercy of others, or fate, or luck, or chance; certainly that is what most people on this planet live by. But once you start to see the Law of Attraction in operation, you ultimately come to understand that there is no such thing as a victim; never has been, never will be.

There is no good luck, bad luck, good fortune or coincidence. There is no destiny, fate or providence. There is no big judge in the sky keeping score on how right or wrong you've been. There is no karma from past lives nor penance.

That's all victim stuff. And there is not a victim among us, only co-creators in thought and feeling, powerful magnets attracting like bees to honey the matching frequency of our ever-flowing vibrations."
—**Lynn Grabhorn, Excuse Me, Your Life Is Waiting, p.23-24**

"Every person, all the events of your life are there because you have drawn them there. What you choose to do with them is up to you."
- **Richard Bach, author of Jonathan Livingston Seagull and Illusions**

"I wake up in the morning, and I consciously create my day the way I want it to happen. Now, sometimes, because my mind is examining all the things that I need to get done, it takes me a little bit to settle down, and get to the point, of where I'm actually intentionally creating my day. But here's the thing. When I create my day, and out of nowhere, little things happen that are so unexplainable, I know that they are the process or the result of my creation. And the more I do that, the more I build a neural net, in my brain, that I accept that that's possible, gives me the power and the incentive to do it the next day."
- **Dr. Joe Dispenza from the film "What the Bleep Do We know?"**

Getting to Cause (Cause > Effect)

One of the challenges of this concept of becoming "Response-Able" is the idea that if we are to truly move away from the victim mentality, then how do we account for horrible instances of abuse and cruelty, tragedy and horror that really do seem to come from outside ourselves?

> This is not an idea we can easily embrace. It is a discussion we cannot fully bring ourselves to because we are so deeply terrified by the heinous acts in our world, confused by and afraid of the pain and injustice and danger. Yet in the larger context we must at least ask, "Could there be meaning and purpose in them?"
>
> We fear that if we allow that there is purpose, it means we must accept the gross inequities and exonerate the people who perpetuate them. But this idea defies reason. It is a "victim" mentality. Feeling on the other hand the situation is unredeemable and beyond our control leaves us without option. But recognizing the purpose or opportunity in such chaotic events, we can then utilize them to bring change. When we see the larger purpose underlying an event, our understanding aids us in healing the pain and bringing about growth. When we act on that understanding, we learn to trust ourselves.
>
> - Lenedra J. Carroll, The Architecture of All Abundance (pages 282-283), published by New World Libaray, Novato, California 2001

The point for this program is that it is up to us to discern meaning from the events of our lives. By choosing to find a positive purpose in whatever "happened" to us as kids or teenagers or even last week, we can gather the power to change our "now."

So just consider for a moment. Do you want to accept the challenge of owning your experience and thereby becoming empowered to change it or would you rather just blame your "condition" on factors outside of your control?

More on getting to Cause:

Your thoughts have bio-chemical consequences in your body.

Imagine going to the refrigerator and taking out a bowl of perfectly ripe lemons...

The sun is streaming through your kitchen window. And as you take a lemon and a knife and begin to cut through the rind, pungent oils from the lemon skin spray out catching the sun's rays as they mist out that lemon fresh fragrance...

Now cut a nice big wedge out of that lemon and... Take the wedge... and imagine biting into it... can you taste the tart, sour, citrus, lemon juice exploding on your tongue?

Doesn't just thinking about biting into a lemon make your mouth pucker and produce more saliva? I know every time I describe this process to one of my clients or audiences, I definitely get a rush of saliva in my mouth.

Your mind doesn't distinguish between what is experienced and what is imagined.

Studies were done where a person's brain was hooked up to sophisticated sensors. The person then was given something to look at and the neural net lit up in a specific part of the brain. Then the person was asked to close their eyes and imagine the same object. the brain reacted exactly the same way. **(source: What the Bleep Do We Know?)**

So if you are imagining yourself to be fat, your brain will deliver all the chemicals, enzymes, Neuro-peptides etc. that make that a reality. Imagine yourself thin and the same process will begin to deliver a very different reality

It also helps if you:
a. visualize yourself actually getting up off the couch and moving around a bit and
b. stop eating large quantities of crap!).

Ah, but sometimes it's not so simple. Sometimes there are multiple old programs and patterns of thought that sabotage your conscious attempts at "thinking positive" and "doing the right thing".

Later on you will learn how to clear old programs and retrain your brain to give you more and more of what you want.

One thing we can do right away is to start anchoring these concepts internally. One very effective way to do that is through songs. This whole journey for me started out with writing songs. My songs have always been more about transformation and making sense of the world than about your typical teenage love angst. Lately I've been writing songs about NLP!

The next few pages contain lyrics to songs that present this information poetically/musically.

Have you ever gotten a song stuck in your head?

There is actually a part of your brain called the "Rostro-Medial Pre-Frontal Cortex" that is closely linked to physical movement like dance.

The idea is to listen to these songs repeatedly until they are playing in your head even without the CD. You can listen to them free of charge at: www.ItsNotJustAboutTheFood.com

Play them in the car when you're driving around. Play them softly in the background while you are going about your day. Some people play them while they sleep. This is one nearly effortless way to begin to reprogram yourself. It's also supposed to be enjoyable. So if you don't care for my style of music go out and find your own tunes that support positive change.

Snap Out Of It

Something happened that you didn't want to happen
Now you think that everything has turned to crap and
The Universe would like it if you failed…
Don't you think that pattern's just a little stale?

When I hear your story I just can not help but wonder
What was it that you chose to think that tore your heart asunder?
What if you had seen it differently?
Like maybe now at last you could be free?

Refrain: Snap out of it, Snap out of it, Snap out of it baby
             Do you think it would break your face to smile?
             Baby I have seen friendlier crocodiles

Now I'm not saying that your lover didn't hurt you
I'm not saying he or she did not desert you
All I'm saying is **now you get to choose**
Whether you will grow and learn or simply sing the blues

Refrain: Snap out of it, Snap out of it, Snap out of it baby
             Do you think that you're the only one?
             What would it cost for you to have some fun?

Sometimes I wonder what it takes to get you moving
Do you need a shock, a shout, a drug that's proven?
I'm not sure that we will ever know
Meantime, you've been tumbling in the under tow

Refrain: Snap out of it, Snap out of it, Snap out of it baby
             Do you think Rome was built in a day?
             So get to work or go outside and get to play!

Now don't get mad at me for popping your self- pity
Sometimes it feels so good to see the world as shitty
Once I was much whinier than you
'Til someone shoved my nose into a different point of view
And I had simply had to…

Refrain: Snap out of it, Snap out of it, Snap out of it baby
             Did you lose the wind from out your sails?
             What would you do if you knew you could not fail?

Change is everywhere you look, you're gonna find it.
Change your job, your look, your cover, change your mind, it
Changes your thoughts which change the way you feel
Pay attention baby cause your thoughts are real.

Refrain:

Commentary: This song is about taking charge of your emotional states. I don't always want to hear this song but it does snap me out of any funk I may get into. (yes I still get into funks now and then. But a hell of a lot less than I used to. I spent most of my life (until recently) wallowing in one down state or another. This program is all about helping you to "snap out of" whatever patterns have gotten you to where you are now...

Mark Shepard, NLPT—Master Practitioner & Trainer of NLP, Hypnosis & Time Line Therapy™:
Rapid Results for Individual and Organizational Empowerment & Transformation
ItsNotJustAboutTheFood.com Copyright 2003, 2004, 2005, 2013, 2014 by Mark Shepard All Rights Reserved

Roll Your Rock Away

You could believe in Santa Clause
Yet still not believe in yourself
You could pause because
You're afraid of your turn
In the urn up on the living room shelf
You could have a brand new set of Ginsu knives
You could have more good luck than
An alley cat's got lives
You could out deal the devil in the dark of night
While you scan the future with your second sight
But you got to roll your rock away

You could dance to the beat
Of a different drummer
While you drive down the street
In your bright red Hummer
You might look hot on the beach this summer
Or be the coolest dude in a crowd of cucumbers
You could talk a dog off a meat wagon
Convince Austin Powers to give up shagging
Or Sell snow to the city of Buffalo
As part of your own reality T.V. Show
But you got to roll your rock away.

You may have the cleanest house in Babylon
Or the best tasting salt in Gomorra
You may be the latest prophet reciting
From the Bible, the Koran,
The Wall St. Journal, or the Torah
You can get yourself a groovy guru
And a magical mantra to mutter
Or you may prefer modern scientific Voodoo
As you hit the links with your carbon fiber putter
You got to roll your rock away.

Bridge:
Would you dare to take my hand?
Let me show you your own Promised Land
It begins when you choose to see
Yourself the way you want to be…
(You got to roll your rock away)

You could be drowning in the desert
Thirsty in the pouring rain
You might be wondering
When someone's gonna finally explain
Why you can lead a horse to water
You might even get your horse to drink
You can lead a man to knowledge
But I'll be damned if you can make him think
He's got to roll his own rock away
You got to roll your rock away…

Commentary: This is a hopefully humorous approach to getting the concept across that it is up to us to create what we want in our lives.

I can't lose weight for you...That's the rock you've got to roll away…

I can coach you and reconnect you with the many resources you have. I can even loan you a lever and a fulcrum so that it's a lot easier to move the rock than you thought.

But...it's your rock and ultimately it's up to you to make the changes you want in your life now.

Mark Shepard, NLPT—Master Practitioner & Trainer of NLP, Hypnosis & Time Line Therapy™:
Rapid Results for Individual and Organizational Empowerment & Transformation
ItsNotJustAboutTheFood.com Copyright 2003, 2004, 2005, 2013, 2014 by Mark Shepard All Rights Reserved

On The Cause Way

You can be who you choose to be
You have everything that you need
To allow yourself to set yourself free
You may not think you are free
You may think you need some kind of key
To unlock the door that isn't there…

If you focus hard enough
It's on the floor with the other stuff
But you must bend to pick it up
You can turn it upside down
You can turn it all around
You can even choose to leave it on the ground

Refrain:
There's a light out on the causeway
Not everyone can see it glow
You may dream you're wide-awake
Don't you know that's how you'll know?

What you see is what you create
From the thoughts you think that dominate
As you fix or change your state
What can now be pre-supposed?
Are we parts or are we whole?
The most flexible has the most control

Refrain:

You may look up or glance across
You may look down to feel a loss
Or you may choose to look inside
You may remember to the left
While you create your future right
Exactly how, you do it best…

Refrain:

Commentary: This song is full of concepts that support the process of moving from the victim side (being at effect of something outside yourself) to the cause side of the equation (where you have the power to change your life).

This song also has several "embedded" poetic references to NLP eye patterns as well as the pre-suppositions of NLP.

Eyes on the Horizon

Dare to live your life lighter
Tune it up like a pow-wow drum
Watch yourself getting brighter
Shine out louder than the noon day sun
Feel your clothes getting looser
Now that you are freely moving
Focus in on the good stuff
As you get yourself to really grooving
Catch a glimpse of the true you, And not just because Simon says…

Refrain: (repeat 1st line after each other line)
Keep your eyes on the horizon, your awareness at the edge
And the next time you blink you will have some new knowledge…
You have everything you need to take your next step now…
You have everything you need to get yourself to "Wow"…
Keep your eyes on the horizon…

Dare to laugh yourself silly
At all the old victim dramas
Shake yourself like a wet dog shedding
All the self inflicted traumas
Shape shift to a new you
It can even be fun to do
Take a trip to a new view
Without a ticket to Katmandu
Take a look at the true you, And not just because Simon says…

Refrain:

Wake up to the new thing
Wake up hear the song birds singing
Wake up to better, whether
You want to be here or there…
Give voice to the inside story
Let go of the obligatory
Routines so you can be free
To live impeccably
Take a look at the true you, And not just because Simon says

Refrain:

Commentary: This song is actually a "wide-awake" hypnotic induction. It's sets the stage for all we will be learning. It is also a great tool for reinforcing all the changes you've begun to make. Might I suggest to you that you play this song over and over and over and over and over and over and over and over?

Chapter Five
Taking Back Your Life And Body

Mark Shepard, NLPT—Master Practitioner & Trainer of NLP, Hypnosis & Time Line Therapy™:
Rapid Results for Individual and Organizational Empowerment & Transformation
ItsNotJustAboutTheFood.com Copyright 2003, 2004, 2005, 2013, 2014 by Mark Shepard All Rights Reserved

Steps to taking back your life and body

1. **Take "Response-Ability"** for where you are and "get to cause". If you created this, then you can create something better. By the way, this is NOT blame. Responsibility literally means "being able to respond." What is it that you want to create?

2. **Educate yourself.** Learn how to run your brain and communicate effectively with your unconscious mind so you can begin to manifest the kind of body and life you want now. Learn about your body and how to better support your health nutritionally. Model other people who have successfully done what you want to do.

3. **Expand Your perceptions**. Eliminate old routines and patterns of behavior. Many books say you should "change." This is "how to change".

4. **Clarify Your Values.** What is most important to you?

5. **Focus on what you want.** Create a powerfully vivid fully sensory visualization of what you want. Write it down, record it, engrave it on your being.

6. **Clear up** the **past.** Stalk and release negative emotions, dis-empowering beliefs and limiting decisions not consistent with what you want.

7. **Program your future** by inserting your goals into your future timeline

8. **Align** your **Thoughts** with your **Goals**

9. **Take Action**. Play everything at **100%**.

10. **Get support. Reinforce** the positive results.

11. **Get support Reinforce** the positive results.

12. **Get Support. Reinforce** the positive results.

13. **Get Support. Reinforce** the positive results.

14. **Get Support. Reinforce** the positive results.

15. **Get Support Reinforce** the positive results.

Mark Shepard, NLPT—Master Practitioner & Trainer of NLP, Hypnosis & Time Line Therapy™:
Rapid Results for Individual and Organizational Empowerment & Transformation
ItsNotJustAboutTheFood.com Copyright 2003, 2004, 2005, 2013, 2014 by Mark Shepard All Rights Reserved

Take "Response-Ability" for where you are.

If you created this, Then you can create something better. By the way, this is NOT blame. You've already been beating up on yourself enough haven't you?

Consider this: Who you are now is the sum of all the thoughts, memories, perceptions, visualizations, self-talk and past programming you've been running all your life. If that has gotten you an unsatisfactory result then it's time to do something different isn't it?

Some key beliefs you need to program into your unconscious mind: (these come from the "pre-suppositions of NLP")

a. There is no failure. Only feedback.
b. Everyone is doing the best they can with the resources they perceive to be available
c. Everyone has all the resources they need in order to get the results they want (even if they don't yet perceive that they have those resources).
d. In order to access our additional resources we need to expand our perception enough to become aware of them.

Three steps to success:
In the context of losing weight and transforming yourself into a lean, high energy, healthy person we need to:

> Engaging in a diet in order to fit society's perceptions of body image is clearly not effective. At the source of many unsuccessful diets are the unhealthy, critical feelings we have toward our bodies and our food. These feelings set up an antagonistic relationship with what we eat. Every mouthful is regretted, judged. In the entertainment industry, I meet many men and women who feel guilty with every bite of food they take. That is not an intent that generates a successful wave—it washes back into the body as a disturbing fear-based frequency.
> —Lenedra J. Carrol, The Architecture of All Abundance,

1. Address old past patterns and programming. Heal the hurt parts of our lives.
2. Learn how to run our brain and take charge of our internal representations so that we are in control of what food means to us and aware of how we are using food to medicate the hurt parts of our lives.
3. Understand the science and physiology behind why diets have failed us and will always fail us. Extensive research as well as practical experience proves **diets actually cause us to retain fat and become less energetic and more sluggish.** Once we understand this we can use our tools of transformation to literally reset our weight regulating mechanism, as well as to change numerous other small and large behavioral and metabolic programs.

What is a healthy diet* anyway?

Consider this, our early ancestors lived on a diet of meat, fish, nuts, vegetables, roots and fruits. Every once in a while they would stumble upon a bee hive and get some honey. In the anthropological record, tooth decay did not exist until hunters and gatherers settled down and started to grow corn and other grain crops.

There is a lot of anthropological evidence to indicate that a high proportion of a hunter gatherer's diet was made up of vegetables and a moderate amount of meat.

There are other benefits of eating a lot of vegetables.
• You can eat as much as you want.
• They contain healthy amounts of fiber and anti–oxidants.
• They are cheaper and more readily available year round than ever before.

Meat and other high protein foods like fish and nuts also contain fat which contrary to our "Fat Phobic" society is actually a much better thing to eat than refined flour, and simple sugars.

A moderate amount of healthy fat helps the body to feel full sooner (as does bulk). Next time you want a snack? Eat an avocado with a bit of Olive oil on it. It contains the "healthy" kind of fat and is a good source of fiber. You feel full. Another benefit of high protein sources of food is that you need protein to build healthy muscle tissue. Muscle cells burn more energy than fat cells. You will be building muscle as you start to move more.

But the best and healthiest diet is the one that you feel good eating. I tried a macrobiotic diet once that was full of vegetables and complex carbohydrates like brown rice...my system did not like it!

I had no energy. I felt bloated and lethargic...it wasn't until someone suggested I cut out most carbs for a while that I discovered I didn't need as much sleep, stopped feeling drowsy after lunch. Had a lot more energy.

I can't tell you what your body burns best. But I would be willing to bet you know already. In case you don't, use your food log to keep track of how you feel after eating different foods.

For example, after eating Pizza, do you feel like taking a walk or taking a nap? I usually feel like going and lying down after pizza! For a long time! So I eat it very, very rarely. The taste sensation isn't usually worth the sluggishness.

It seems that the only thing all the experts agree on is that refined carbohydrates and the kinds of modified hydrogenated fats such as those used in fast food deep fryers and most snack foods are bad.

Fresh natural foods are good. I have a personal goal of eating some veggies with every meal (even breakfast). And in my book potatoes are not on the list. They are very high on the simple carb list. (I do eat them every once in a while now, but much, much less than the days when I had potatoes at almost every meal).

So LISTEN TO YOUR BODY.

Try a couple weeks of low carbs with a lot of veggies..

Try a couple weeks of complex carbs, whole grains with a lot of veggies...keep track of how you feel.

One couple I know are both in pretty good shape. He eats pretty much everything but rarely does dessert. She is a vegetarian and eats a bit of chocolate...They both are extremely physically fit and active...different diets* work for different people. Neither one of them count calories or limit their portions.

*by the way "diet" here simply means the stuff you eat. Not some sadistic torture mechanism that fools your body into thinking you are suffering from a famine(a.k.a. "Reduced Calorie Diet")!

Mark Shepard, NLPT—Master Practitioner & Trainer of NLP, Hypnosis & Time Line Therapy™:
Rapid Results for Individual and Organizational Empowerment & Transformation
ItsNotJustAboutTheFood.com Copyright 2003, 2004, 2005, 2013, 2014 by Mark Shepard All Rights Reserved

Why Reduced Calorie Diets Don't Work

Basically reduced calorie diets don't work because they make your body think it's starving. So you body responds by making internal adjustments to burn more efficiently and even store more fat. Inside one of the oldest parts of our brains is an information center known as the Hypothalamus. it's job is to regulate all kinds of functions in your body. One of the main functions of this part of your brain is called the "Weight Regulating Mechanism"

Pioneering weight loss researchers Dennis W Remington, MD, A. Garth Fisher, PhD and Edward A. Parent, PhD identify something called the "Weight Regulating Mechanism".

The Weight Regulating Mechanism consists of three parts: **your appetite, your metabolism and your set point.**

Your set point is a lot like the thermostat found in most houses. It is set for a certain temperature and if the temperature drops below a certain point the heat turns on. The furnace stops when the house warms up to a certain temperature.

The set point is like that. You decide to go on a reducing diet and essentially you alert the system that there is less energy coming in.

So your set point flashes on and calls for more.

You haven't told your set point that it should just be set lower, its no big deal.

There is no famine in the land! But your set point doesn't know this!

It calls for more food.

So your appetite kicks in and starts hollering at you to shove more fuel in the furnace.

You can hold out for a while but eventually (like when you hold your breath and reach a point when you absolutely must breathe) there is a point when your unconscious survival mechanism takes over and you break down and start binge eating.

Right?

I don't know if you've ever been in a house where the thermostat wasn't quite right?

In order to get 68 degrees you had to set it on 80? Well that's what your set point does, it doesn't want this to happen again so it sets itself higher so your metabolism slows down at the same time your appetite is calling for you to eat more. And, just in case this is a big famine, your body ends up storing more fat.

Mark Shepard, NLPT—Master Practitioner & Trainer of NLP, Hypnosis & Time Line Therapy™:
Rapid Results for Individual and Organizational Empowerment & Transformation
ItsNotJustAboutTheFood.com Copyright 2003, 2004, 2005, 2013, 2014 by Mark Shepard All Rights Reserved

The other thing that happens is your weight regulating mechanism slows down your resting metabolism.

This is like going around and closing all the windows in the house and putting up heavy insulated draperies and insulating the walls.

So now the system is even more efficient and even more tuned to survive the non existent famine.

Put this all together and your reduced calorie diet has literally caused you to be miserable, beat up on yourself because you couldn't stick to it, feel like you're starving and totally confuse your body into thinking that it should actually conserve more energy rather than start to burn the plentiful stored energy that we call FAT.

I can't tell what to do but I know this. Reduced Calorie, Low Fat Diets don't work.

You probably know this too...How many diets have you been on in your life?

List all the diets you've been on in the space below:

_____

_____

_____

_____

_____

_____

_____

_____

_____

_____

_____

_____

_____

_____

_____

_____

Mark Shepard, NLPT—Master Practitioner & Trainer of NLP, Hypnosis & Time Line Therapy™:
Rapid Results for Individual and Organizational Empowerment & Transformation
ItsNotJustAboutTheFood.com Copyright 2003, 2004, 2005, 2013, 2014 by Mark Shepard All Rights Reserved

Are You Eating Enough Fat Lately?

In his book the Fat Fallacy, Dr. Will Clower, (published by Three Rivers Press, NY, 2002) makes a pretty good case for the fact that one key factor in the high rate of Obesity in Americans is the past 30 year trend towards a low fat diet.

Clower is a neurophysiologist who took a two year assignment in France. While there, he and his family tucked right in to the sumptuous French diet that included plenty of butter, cream and full fat cheeses. They all lost weight!

His mom joined them for a while and before leaving the states resigned herself to just enjoying the French food without worrying about how much she would "gain". She packed lots of baggy sweat suits and literally forgot about dieting. When she returned home she "had gone from a size 12-begging-to-be-a-size-14 to a size 6, dancing around our living room floor with her arms up in the air like she had just won the lottery—in my wife's blue jeans!" p. 14

One of your first assignments is to get a copy of this book and read it.

I would never suggest you suddenly start to eat this way, that decision is yours alone. I do however want you to consider just how much better you life would be if you were enjoying your food and focusing on creating a balanced, healthy lifestyle that included more of the attitude of the French and Italians who spend more time enjoying their food and a lot less time running around like crazy people, stuffing fast food into their mouths while they race from one thing to another...

In my own personal food plan, I eat a lot of vegetables either steamed or sautéed in coconut oil. I drink a café late every morning with 1/2 & 1/2 instead of milk. I eat the healthiest meats I can (grass fed, free range, natural and organic).

I make sure I get plenty of healthy fats like coconut oil, olive oil and fish oil supplements. I eat a bit of raw milk cheese. I take nuts and veggies with me for snacks. I also eat ice cream about once a month or so and some desserts in moderation. And I feel pretty damn good. I also have lost about 15 pounds and gone down a pants size since I last tried to include significant amounts of carbs in my diet.

Again, that's what seems to work for me. Reading this book is one step in opening your mind to new ideas so that you can begin to change your life in a way that is as easy and effortless as possible...

The second book that is important in understanding the role of healthy fats in our diets is "Healthy Fats For Life" by Lorna R. Vanderhaeghe & Karlene Karst, published by John Wiley and Sons Canada, Ltd. 2004

Not only do the "good fats" help in losing weight and feeling better, they can be a factor in prevention and treatment of many other health conditions as well.

Research into the "right Fat" diet has been conflicting. We have been told that margarine is better for us than butter. Then some scientists did a complete about face and we were advised that we should eat butter instead of margarine. Many of us stopped eating eggs because doctors told us they added to our high cholesterol. Then a decade later nutritionists said, "Eggs are good for you and have little effect on cholesterol." Fats are bad for us is another myth perpetuated by those who fail to understand how all the different types of fats affect the body. Lumping all fat into the same category has caused the disease scales to rise.

Thousands of studies worldwide,...provide solid evidence that not only are certain fats not bad for us, but they are essential for life. Extra virgin olive oil, organic flaxseed oil, coconut butter, coconut oil, coconut milk, borage, evening primrose, fish oils, butter and CLA provide amazing healing properties. These marvelous healing fats reduce our risk of heart disease and diabetes, help us burn fat, oil arthritic joints, prevent depression, manufacture our hormones improve our skin, boost our immune system and so much more.—from the introduction p. vii

Here's the very least you need to know:

The Good: <u>Short chain saturates</u> found in butter, coconut oil and palm kernel oil do not clog arteries, nor do they cause heart disease. Rather, they are easily digested and a good source of fuel for energy....

The Not-So-Bad: <u>Medium-chain saturates</u> are found in several different foods, but the highest content (just as in short chain saturates) is also found in palm kernel and coconut oils, and they are not associated with increasing cholesterol levels or the occurrence of heart disease.

The Bad: <u>Long chain saturates</u> are the "bad" fats associated with raising LDL (the bad cholesterol), lowering HDL (the good cholesterol) and the increasing risk of heart disease. Long chain saturates are also a by-product of hydrogenation, a process that turns a liquid fat (at room temperature into a sold and is employed in the manufacture of most margarines and shortening. Long chain saturates are also abundantly present in restaurant fried foods, junk food, packaged baked goods and processed foods. Hydrogenation or partial hydrogenation also distorts the fatty acids into a more poisonous form. (p.3-4)

It doesn't take a scientist to figure out that we Americans eat a lot of foods that contain the bad fats. Almost every packaged food item we buy at the grocery store from microwave popcorn, to cookies contains an alarming amount of these bad fats. This is vital information for you to know if you are serious about getting fit and healthy.

Read this book. What you learn might save your life.

White Fat vs. Brown Fat:

Researchers also discovered that there were two different kinds of fat in our bodies. "White" or "storage" fat which the body creates as a storage for lean times and "Brown" or "active" fat which provides fuel to be actively burned by the muscles.

Lean, high energy people seem to have more of the Brown fat.
Obese and overweight people have less of it and a lot more of the white fat.

For our purposes here, we will be visualizing an increase in Brown fat as well as little fat molecules being steadily fed into the fiery furnace of our muscles to be burned easily and effortlessly...

Brown fat is metabolically active fat that surrounds our organs, cushioning the blood vessels and spinal column....this is the type of fat burned in the body to create heat....White fat is the insulating layer of fat just beneath the skin that buffers us from the cold and stores calories....Thin people have active brown fat while overweight individuals have dormant brown fat. "Healthy Fats For Life" p.28

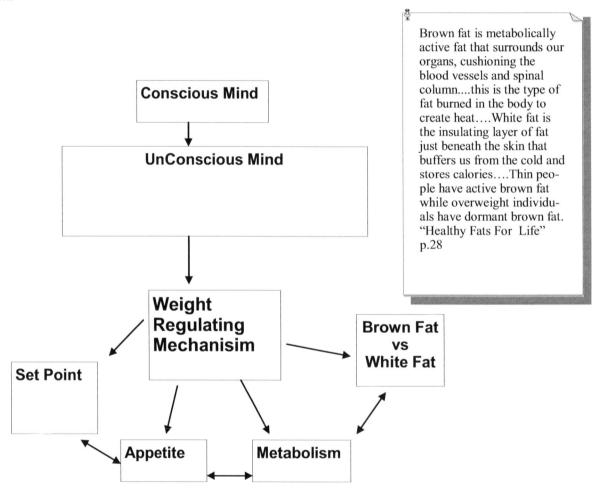

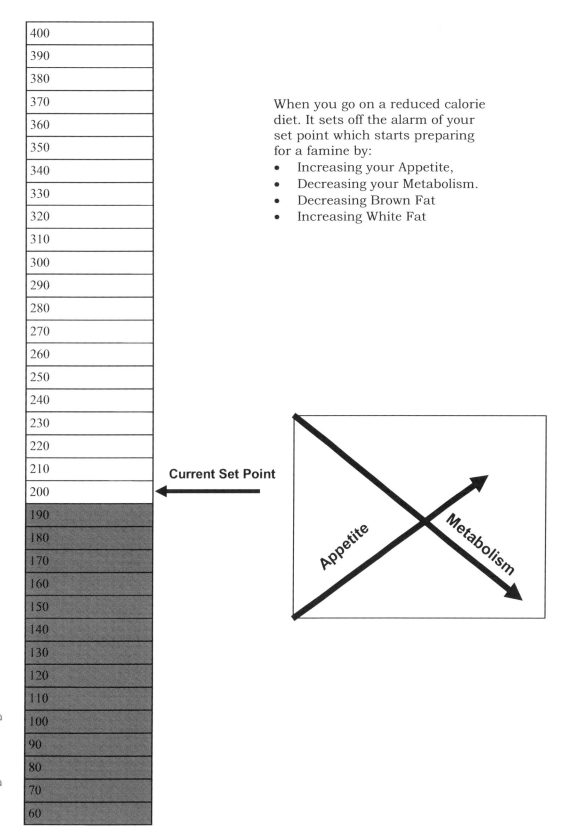

When you go on a reduced calorie diet. It sets off the alarm of your set point which starts preparing for a famine by:

- Increasing your Appetite,
- Decreasing your Metabolism.
- Decreasing Brown Fat
- Increasing White Fat

Mark Shepard, NLPT—Master Practitioner & Trainer of NLP, Hypnosis & Time Line Therapy™:
Rapid Results for Individual and Organizational Empowerment & Transformation
ItsNotJustAboutTheFood.com Copyright 2003, 2004, 2005, 2013, 2014 by Mark Shepard All Rights Reserved

400
390
380
370
360
350
340
330
320
310
300
290
280
270
260
250
240
230
220
210
200
190
180
170
160
150
140
130
120
110
100
90
80
70
60

Old Set Point ← (at 210)

New Set Point ← (at 190)

Eventual Set Point ← (at 130)

Danger! Danger!

You can affect your weight regulating mechanism by using self hypnosis and visualization to:

- Lower Your set point 5 or ten pounds at a time.
- Increase your movement. Walk more, choose the stairs, wiggle when you sit etc.
- Increase your Metabolism
- Increase Brown Fat
- Decrease White Fat

You can affect your weight regulating mechanism by consciously:

- Choosing better, more nutritious food (cutting out most flour and sugar based foods and making sure you eat enough veggies, protein and healthy fats.)
- Supplementing your food intake with metabolism boosting and appetite soothing fiber rich super-foods so you support yourself on the cellular level.
- Focusing on feeling full sooner. Taking smaller bites. Savoring the flavors. Chewing a bit longer. Leaving food on your plate. Eating regular meals. Taking care of yourself by having healthy food to hold you over in the case of an unusually late meal or unavoidable delay.
- Visualizing yourself the way you want to be. Make sure you see yourself in the picture looking the way you want and imagining the way you want to feel.

Appetite

Metabolism

What does work?

If you want to find out how to be lean, model some lean people who were once overweight. Here is what you will find:

1. They have reprogrammed themselves to have high metabolisms. They burn off energy even when sitting "still".

2. Lean people actually don't sit very still even when they are sitting. They wiggle, they shift their positions, they fidget. They do that thing with their legs you know their heel is up in the air and their legs are going a mile a minute? If you don't do that, start now!

3. They move a lot in general.

4. They live interesting, active lives where they are passionate about what they are doing for work and play.

5. They spend a significant amount of time outdoors walking, working, playing sports, gardening, sailing, biking, hiking, building stuff, playing with their kids. They watch less TV than the average overweight person.

6. They don't fight for the parking spaces right near the door of the store! They park their cars farther out. They are impatient with elevators and will just as often take the stairs instead of standing there waiting.

7. They actually eat more food because their bodies are tuned to burning and "wasting" energy.

8. In their childhood response to unpleasant or traumatic events they tended to "protect themselves by "running away" and throwing themselves into activities rather than by armoring and numbing themselves or self soothing with food.

9. When something unpleasant or stressful happens in their lives they tend to go "move it off" or do some very physical activity to blow off steam.

10. They rarely, if ever, eat at a fast food restaurant.

11. They most likely have reduced or eliminated their intake of empty calories, sweets, desserts, fried foods, grains, processed foods, fruit juices, soda, chips, etc.

"Time motion studies have shown that overweight people move less and use less energy than thin people even when doing simple chores like making a bed. The average thin person will move around the bed 7 times while the overweight person tends to accomplish more from the same position… it is as if the overweight persons weight regulating mechanism is telling their body to move more slowly, work more efficiently and rest more often."

– Neuropsychology of Weight Control—Dennis W. Remington, MD, A. Garth Fisher, PhD, Edward A. Parent, PhD. SyberVision Systems,

Mark Shepard, NLPT—Master Practitioner & Trainer of NLP, Hypnosis & Time Line Therapy™:
Rapid Results for Individual and Organizational Empowerment & Transformation
ItsNotJustAboutTheFood.com Copyright 2003, 2004, 2005, 2013, 2014 by Mark Shepard All Rights Reserved

What doesn't work?

If you want to find out how to be overweight, model some overweight people.

Here is what you will find.

1. They have tried and failed at many, many diets and as a result are angry, frustrated and discouraged.
2. They have slow metabolisms. And make internal pictures of themselves as even fatter than they actually are.
3. They tend to sit for long periods of time with almost no wiggling or fidgeting.
4. They have bought into the "low fat" foods industry without realizing "low fat" usually means high sugar content or a bunch of chemicals.
5. When they do move they will move as efficiently as possible and tend to move and walk slower than their lean counterparts
6. They tend to dislike their jobs, are frustrated with their relationships, are bored with their lives or so busy, and stressed out that they can barely make it through the day. For many, the couch and TV is the only thing they can force themselves to do at the end of the day.
7. They are really good at beating up on themselves. They tend to get disappointed easily and have a tendency towards depression and pessimism.
8. In their childhood response to unpleasant or traumatic events they tended to "protect themselves by armoring and numbing themselves.
9. Many of them had severely critical or dysfunctional families and have numerous limiting beliefs about themselves, low self esteem, negative self talk, and internal representations about themselves and often can't even imagine themselves lean, and healthy.
10. They use food to soothe or "medicate" their unresolved emotional pain or frustration in relationships and disappointments.
11. They use food to reward themselves.
12. They think about food all the time except when they are actually eating at which point they tend to "trance out" and have no conscious awareness of how much they've eaten or how full they are.

The mind and body are so interconnected that we must address the physical as well as the emotional aspects of the person. How do we do that?

1. Stop "dieting" and eat a balanced variety of good nutritious food in moderation. Decrease sugar, wheat and corn based foods. Increase vegetables and healthy fats like Coconut Oil, Olive Oil, Macadamia nut oil. Increase, water intake, supplements that support healthy cellular nutrition and metabolism boosting...
2. Release negative emotions, limiting beliefs and decisions from the past.
3. Interrupt habitual negative behavior patterns and install more effective behavioral strategies on the unconscious level.
4. Monitor old self talk and begin to install new linguistic "afformations"
5. Adjust the weight regulating mechanism through hypnosis, self hypnosis, creative visualization, and consistent, moderate, low impact exercise that incorporates "interval" training.
6. Keep track of successes and increase positive reinforcement of changes made.

Mark Shepard, NLPT—Master Practitioner & Trainer of NLP, Hypnosis & Time Line Therapy™:
Rapid Results for Individual and Organizational Empowerment & Transformation
ItsNotJustAboutTheFood.com Copyright 2003, 2004, 2005, 2013, 2014 by Mark Shepard All Rights Reserved

WATER
HOW 8 GLASSES A DAY KEEP THE FAT AWAY

Incredible as it may seem, water is quite possibly the single most important catalyst in losing weight and keeping it off. Although most of us take it for granted, water may be the only true "magic potion"
for permanent weight loss.

Water suppresses the appetite naturally and helps the body metabolize stored fat. Studies have shown that a decrease in water intake will cause fat deposits to increase, while an increase in water intake can actually reduce fat deposits.

Here's why: The kidneys can't function properly without enough water. When they don't work to capacity, some of their load is dumped onto the liver.

One of the liver's primary functions is to metabolize stored fat into usable energy for the body. But, if the liver has to do some of the kidney's work, it can't operate at full throttle. As a result, it metabolizes less fat, and more fat remains stored in the body and weight loss stops.

Fluid Retention
Drinking enough water is the best treatment for fluid retention. When the body gets less water, it perceives this as a threat to survival and begins to hold on to every drop. Water is stored in extracellular spaces (outside the cells). This shows up as swollen feet, legs and hands.

Diuretics offer a temporary solution at best. They force out stored water along with some essential nutrients.

Again, the body perceives a threat and will replace the lost water at the first opportunity. Thus, the condition quickly returns.

The best way to overcome the problem of water retention is to give your body what it needs-- plenty of water. Only then will stored water be released.

If you have a constant problem with water retention, excess salt may be to blame. Your body will tolerate sodium only in a certain concentration. The more salt you eat, the more water your system retains to dilute it.

But, getting rid of unneeded salt is easy—just drink more water. As it is forced through the kidneys it takes away excess sodium. Speaking of salt, make sure you are using a high quality sea salt. It contains essential minerals and trace elements that your body needs.

More Benefits:

Water helps to maintain proper muscle tone by giving muscles their natural ability to contract and by preventing dehydration. It also helps to prevent the sagging skin that usually follows weight loss – shrinking cells are buoyed by water, which plumps the skin and leaves it clear, healthy and resilient.

Water helps rid the body of waste. During weight loss, the body has a lot more waste to get rid of – all that metabolized fat must be shed. Again, adequate water helps flush out the waste.

Constipation:
Water can help relieve constipation. When the body gets too little water, it siphons what it needs from internal sources. The colon is one primary source. Result? Constipation. But, when a person drinks enough water, normal bowel function usually returns.
Remarkable Water!

So far, we've discovered some remarkable things about water and weight loss:

- The body will not function properly without enough water and can't metabolize stored fat efficiently.
- Retained water shows up as excess weight.
- To get rid of excess water you must drink more water.
- Drinking water is essential to weight loss.

How much water is enough?

On the average, a person should drink eight (8-ounce) glasses every day; that's about 2 quarts. However, the overweight person needs one additional glass for every 25 pounds of excess weight. The amount you drink also should be increased if you exercise briskly or if the weather is hot and dry.

Water should preferably be cold—it's absorbed into the system more quickly than warm water. And some evidence suggests that drinking cold water can actually help burn calories.

Breakthrough Point

When the body gets the water it needs to function optimally, its fluids are perfectly balanced. When this happens you have reached the "breakthrough point". *What does this mean?*
- Endocrine gland function improves.
- Fluid retention is alleviated, as stored water is lost.
- More fat is used as fuel because the liver is free to metabolize stored fat.
- Natural thirst returns.
- There is a loss of hunger almost overnight.

If you stop drinking enough water your body fluids will be thrown out of balance again, and you may experience fluid retention, unexplained weight gain and loss of thirst.

To remedy the situation you'll have to go back and force another "breakthrough".

Drink plenty of water!!

And while we are talking about drinking things...

You must absolutely positively STOP drinking diet beverages.

They are definitely one of the worst, most toxic things you can put in your body. The artificial sweetners contain "Excito-Toxins" which interact with your brain and body chemistry in an extremely negative way.

Mark Shepard, NLPT—Master Practitioner & Trainer of NLP, Hypnosis & Time Line Therapy™:
Rapid Results for Individual and Organizational Empowerment & Transformation
ItsNotJustAboutTheFood.com Copyright 2003, 2004, 2005, 2013, 2014 by Mark Shepard All Rights Reserved

Have you ever noticed that many really fat people drink diet soda?

Sometimes I just want to ask them, "How's that diet soda working?"

On a personal note: my mother used artificial sweetners for years and years.

She didn't make it past her mid 70's...

My dad who was about the same age as mom, got into health foods back when he was in his 40's. Ironically my mom made teased him about being a "health food nut" for years.

He is now in his 80's and his best friends, Josh and Louise are in their 20's and 30's and extremely fit even for people in their age group.

My dad gives them a run for their money!

He and Josh make beer and raw milk cheeses and yogurt and Kefir and Kim Chee and Saurkraut on a regular basis. He gets up early, stays up late and has energy to burn all day. He swims 3 times a week. He's a volunteer driver for social services. He heats his house with wood, which he still splits and hauls by hand. His stomach is flat. He is as fit as someone many, many years younger. Oh, and I forgot to mention he is an above the knee amputee (from a childhood illness) and walks so well with his prosthetic leg that most people don't know he's got an artificial leg unless he's wearing his shorts!

I share his story because he smoked and drank and ate crap until he was in his forties when a health crisis "woke him up" and he choose to change his way of eating.

And you also must stop drinking fruit juices and regular soda. It is sugar!

You would never sit down an d eat 8 oranges at a time would you? How many oranges are in a single glass of juice?

Drink water! If you absolutely can't stand plain water, a squeeze of lemon or lime can add a bit of zest and excitement.

If it absolutely has to be fizzy, drink seltzer water, (water that has bubbles of air in it not sodium carbonate. Get it? "carbonation" is the result of Sodium! What is sodium? SALT!)

No matter what *your* age, you can begin today to take exquisite care of your body by drinking enough fresh, filtered, clean, clear, pure water.

You'll know you are drinking enough water when your urine is very light yellow or even clear.

Don't believe me?

Check out this book: "Your Body's Many Cries For Water" by by F. Batmanghelidj You might want to also check out one of his other books, "Obesity Cancer & Depression: Their Common Cause & Natural Cure"

Chapter Six
Focusing On Your Progress

Mark Shepard, NLPT—Master Practitioner & Trainer of NLP, Hypnosis & Time Line Therapy™:
Rapid Results for Individual and Organizational Empowerment & Transformation
ItsNotJustAboutTheFood.com Copyright 2003, 2004, 2005, 2013, 2014 by Mark Shepard All Rights Reserved

Taking Response-Ability:
Where You Are Now ?
Where Do You Want To Be?

Today's Date:

_____

Do you have a picture of they way you look slim?

Paste into this workbook along with a picture of you when you were not slim.

If you don't have a slender picture, find a friend who knows their way around Photoshop or some other photo management software. Get them to "slenderize" your picture.

Later we will add additional pictures as you begin to slim down and increase muscle tone.

If you like numbers and charts and all that scientific stuff We've provided them later on in this book. It's up to you how much you want to keep track of. It seems to me you should keep a record so you can gauge and reinforce your progress. The point is to keep track or your progress not punish yourself or add extra stress and hassle to your life.

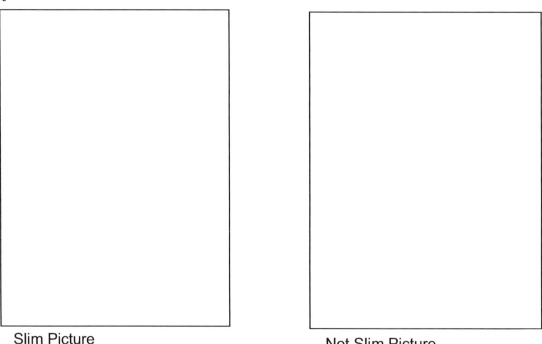

Slim Picture   Not Slim Picture

Mark Shepard, NLPT—Master Practitioner & Trainer of NLP, Hypnosis & Time Line Therapy™:
Rapid Results for Individual and Organizational Empowerment & Transformation
ItsNotJustAboutTheFood.com Copyright 2003, 2004, 2005, 2013, 2014 by Mark Shepard All Rights Reserved

Keys To An Achievable Outcome

1. Stated in the positive. What specifically do I want?

_____

_____

2. Specify Present Situation. Where am I now? (for this question make sure you are Associated, that is you are in the experience looking out through your eyes)

_____

_____

3. Specify Outcome – "What will I see, hear, feel etc. when I have it? (This means that the outcome is viewed as if it were accomplished now. Make it compelling. Then insert it into the future. Be sure that before you insert it into the future that the picture is dissociated, meaning you are looking at yourself from outside of your body as an observer.) Also this is to be stated in the positive making note of what you will experience not what you won't.

_____

_____

4. Evidence Procedure – "How will I know when I have it?"

_____

_____

5. Is it congruently desirable? – "What will this outcome get for me or allow me to do?"

_____

_____

6. Is it Self-Initiated and Maintained? "Is this only for me?" (In other words do you really want this or does someone else in your life think you should want it.)

_____

_____

7. Is it appropriately Contextualized? – "Where, when, how and with whom do I want it?"

_____

_____

Mark Shepard, NLPT—Master Practitioner & Trainer of NLP, Hypnosis & Time Line Therapy™:
Rapid Results for Individual and Organizational Empowerment & Transformation
ItsNotJustAboutTheFood.com Copyright 2003, 2004, 2005, 2013, 2014 by Mark Shepard All Rights Reserved

8. Resources – "What resources do I have now and what resources do I need to get my outcome?"

_____

_____

9. "Have I ever done this before?"_____

10. "Do I know anyone else who has it or has done it?" _____

11. "Just suppose I had it now."_____

12. Check Ecology – "For What purpose do I want this?

_____

13. What will I gain and what will I lose if I have it?" (hint losing could be a good thing in some contexts…)

_____

14. What will happen if I get it?

_____

15. What won't happen if I get it?

_____

16. What will happen if I don't get it?

_____

17. What won't happen if I don't get it?

_____

Notes:

Chapter Seven
Meet Your
Unconscious Mind

Mark Shepard, NLPT—Master Practitioner & Trainer of NLP, Hypnosis & Time Line Therapy™:
Rapid Results for Individual and Organizational Empowerment & Transformation
ItsNotJustAboutTheFood.com Copyright 2003, 2004, 2005, 2013, 2014 by Mark Shepard All Rights Reserved

Meet your Unconscious Mind:

In order to clear unconscious patterns of thought, emotion and behavior it would help to actually know what your unconscious mind is wouldn't it?

Eric Booth in his book, **The Everyday Work of Art: Awakening the Extraordinary in Your Daily Life** (1999, published by Sourcebooks, Inc, P.O. Box 372 Naperville, IL 60566 630-961-3900) gives a great description of your Unconscious Mind.

As a boy his mother took him and his siblings on a trip across the Atlantic Ocean on a German freighter.

As he explored the ship there always seemed to be one grizzled old sailor who was everywhere, silently obeying the orders of the Captain.

Because he has remarkably skinny legs, the family affectionately began calling him "Skinny Legs".

If Eric explored the engine room, there was skinny legs. If he climbed up to the bridge where the ship was steered, there was Skinny Legs alert at the helm.

No matter where he went on the ship, there was Skinny Legs quietly doing his job.

In many ways your unconscious mind is like that. Unfortunately there are certain ways we have to communicate with your unconscious mind so that it clearly gets the message.

We have to speak In positive terms. This is not just because it's "Nice" to be positive. Your Unconscious mind has difficulty processing negatives. For example, you would never say to your Labrador Retriever, "Don't Come!" if you wanted it to stay. You would just tell it to "stay."

> In order to get what you want, first, clear the Unconscious Blocks, Negative Emotions, and Limiting Decisions/ Beliefs That you are using to **create your current reality**.
>
> Then, program your future free of the old baggage...so you can focus on what you <u>do</u> want, instead of on what you <u>don't</u> want.

The conscious mind can handle negatives and we often talk a lot about what we don't want. This has the unfortunate result of programming yourself for failure and disappointment because your unconscious mind only gets what it is you are focusing on.

For example: if a lion was chasing you, you would need to know that and focus on not being eaten for a moment. But then, in order to stay alive, you would have to focus on getting to safety.

If you paid <u>too</u> much attention to the lion.............Gulp!

Another of my favorite analogies for your unconscious mind is that of a powerful and beautiful horse.

Your conscious mind would be the horse trainer.

If the horse trainer is a "horse whisperer" the horse will willingly do any number of behaviors that it might not choose to do on it's own.

But if the horse trainer is cruel or ignorant and tries to force the horse to do something it doesn't want to do, well who is more powerful? The horse or the human?

The horse could easily kick or bite or even crush the trainer.

The point is that your unconscious mind is incredibly powerful. But it is not a logical thinker. It is more animal-like than your conscious mind. The logical reasons to lose weight and get fit work just fine for your conscious mind but may not get translated appropriately to your unconscious.

So that's a significant piece of how this work is different. Unlike a diet which depends on conscious mind "will power." In our program we enlist the help of your powerful unconscious mind to get you where you want to be faster, better easier.

Mark Shepard, NLPT—Master Practitioner & Trainer of NLP, Hypnosis & Time Line Therapy™:
Rapid Results for Individual and Organizational Empowerment & Transformation
ItsNotJustAboutTheFood.com Copyright 2003, 2004, 2005, 2013, 2014 by Mark Shepard All Rights Reserved

YOUR UNCONSCIOUS MIND...

1. **Stores your memories.**

2. **Generates and manages your emotions.**

3. **Organizes all memories.**
   Time Line
   Gestalt

4. **Represses memories with unresolved negative emotion.**

5. **Presents repressed memories for "resolution."**
   (and to release emotions)

6. **Keeps repressed emotions repressed for protection.**

7. **Runs the body.**
   Has a blueprint:
   of body now
   of perfect health- function of the higher self

8. **Preserves the body.**
   Maintains the integrity of the body

Mark Shepard, NLPT—Master Practitioner & Trainer of NLP, Hypnosis & Time Line Therapy™:
Rapid Results for Individual and Organizational Empowerment & Transformation
ItsNotJustAboutTheFood.com Copyright 2003, 2004, 2005, 2013, 2014 by Mark Shepard All Rights Reserved

Your Unconscious Mind (continued)

9. **Is A Highly Moral Being**.

10. **Likes To Follow Directions and wants to serve you.**

11. **Controls and maintains all perceptions.**

    Regular (5 senses)

    Telepathic

    Receives and transmits to the conscious mind.

12. **Generates, stores, distributes and transmits "energy."**

13. **Responds with instinct and habit.**

14. **Needs repetition for long term projects.**

15. **Is Programmed to continually seek more and more.**

    Always more to discover

16. **Does not need parts to function.**

17. **Is Symbolic.**

    Uses and responds to symbols

18. **Takes everything personally.**

19. **Works on the principle of least effort.**

    Path of least resistance

20. **Does not process negatives.**

```
Note to "Skinny
Legs" (a.k.a. Your Uncon-
scious Mind):
```

- Turn off TV.
- Go for a walk. Breathe.
- Move.
- Breathe!
- Enjoy life.
- "Lighten up!"
- Release the stored energy we call "fat".
- Build muscle.
- Increase Metabolism.
- Burn off excess stored energy.
- Create heat.
- Create movement.
- Decrease appetite. Lower set point.
- Eat meals sitting down.
- When eating focus on the flavors and textures and smells of the food.
- Enjoy!
- Drink plenty of water throughout the day.
- Take small bites.
- Chew your food thoroughly.
- Take a new bite only after fully swallowing what was already in mouth.
- Feel full sooner.
- Feel satisfied longer.
- Praise yourself.
- Get out and play.
- Focus on what you want.
- Express appreciation to your body for all it allows you to do and experience...

```
Repeat as necessary...
```

Mark Shepard, NLPT—Master Practitioner & Trainer of NLP, Hypnosis & Time Line Therapy™:
Rapid Results for Individual and Organizational Empowerment & Transformation
ItsNotJustAboutTheFood.com Copyright 2003, 2004, 2005, 2013, 2014 by Mark Shepard All Rights Reserved

Chapter 8
Hypnosis
And Your
Unconscious...
Mind

Mark Shepard, NLPT—Master Practitioner & Trainer of NLP, Hypnosis & Time Line Therapy™:
Rapid Results for Individual and Organizational Empowerment & Transformation
<u>ItsNotJustAboutTheFood.com</u> Copyright 2003, 2004, 2005, 2013, 2014 by Mark Shepard All Rights Reserved

Hypnosis

Now that you've met your unconscious mind, let's learn more about hypnosis and what we can and cannot expect from our new friend.

As I mentioned before, your unconscious mind does not process negatives.

Here's another example. Right now. **Don't think of a blue tree**.

Bet you thought of a blue tree! You did didn't you? Me too.

So if you don't want to eat a certain food, telling yourself not to is literally programming yourself for failure. It would be more helpful to focus on what you want yourself to be wanting. For example, instead of saying "Don't eat the cake!", tell yourself something more useful like, "Forget the cake! let's have a piece of fruit. Or let's go for a walk."

If you want to get up off the couch and exercise do you think it would be more helpful to imagine that great, healthy glow you feel during or after the exercise or do you focus on how soft and comfy the couch is?

The other important thing most people don't know about hypnosis is that **you can't be hypnotized to do something you do not want to do.** It may look that way on TV or in the movies or even with a stage hypnotist. But the reality is if you don't want to exercise I can't "make" you want to exercise. If you want to exercise then I can help you reinforce that desire and teach you how to turn up the volume and make your internal representation of exercise big and bright and appealing.

Some new clients often express a bit of fear that they will "go under" hypnosis and "lose control". Again that's the way things are portrayed in the movies. Most people just feel relaxed. And anyone who has ever been mesmerized by the highway or lost in a good book or totally carried away by a great movie, has already been hypnotized and is familiar with the way trance feels.

Essentially hypnosis is about setting aside your busy, fidgety, compulsive, over thinking , "conscious" mind (Will power) and talking directly to your calm, simple, powerful, results oriented unconscious mind (Imagination).

In a contest between your "Will" and your "Imagination", **Imagination always wins**.

Mark Shepard, NLPT—Master Practitioner & Trainer of NLP, Hypnosis & Time Line Therapy™:
Rapid Results for Individual and Organizational Empowerment & Transformation
ItsNotJustAboutTheFood.com Copyright 2003, 2004, 2005, 2013, 2014 by Mark Shepard All Rights Reserved

Quantum Linguistics:

With these questions we begin to "engage" your unconscious mind in the process of solving your current challenge. Please answer these questions as best you can either on your own or along with the audio recording. Make sure you have a quiet place to work undisturbed for a 30-60 minute block of time. Do your best to ask these questions of your unconscious mind. How? Just relax and drop the question in. Then notice whatever pops to the surface first. Write that down...Try to capture whatever thoughts and images float up first without judging or editing or fretting or fussing...Just trust

1. What was the Problem?

2. How has this problem's presence affected you?

3. What has this problem cost you? What else?

4. What has it cost you that you are pretending not to recognize?

5. What was the cause of this problem (behaviors actually performed by you or beliefs you hold)? When did you choose to have this situation be created? Why? Ask your unconscious mind.

6. How do you want life to be instead?

7. What will this new behavior gain for you? (what else?)

8. What else will happen as a result of this new behavior that you are not thinking of?

Mark Shepard, NLPT—Master Practitioner & Trainer of NLP, Hypnosis & Time Line Therapy™:
Rapid Results for Individual and Organizational Empowerment & Transformation
ItsNotJustAboutTheFood.com Copyright 2003, 2004, 2005, 2013, 2014 by Mark Shepard All Rights Reserved

9. What else will happen as a result of this new behavior that you were pretending not to recognize the need for?

10. What could you have done instead that would have produced the desired results?

11. Have you ever done that? or have you ever known anyone who has done that?

12. What resources do you need that would get you the desired outcomes and prevent the problem from existing in the future?

Mark Shepard, NLPT—Master Practitioner & Trainer of NLP, Hypnosis & Time Line Therapy™:
Rapid Results for Individual and Organizational Empowerment & Transformation
ItsNotJustAboutTheFood.com Copyright 2003, 2004, 2005, 2013, 2014 by Mark Shepard All Rights Reserved

13. Is there anything your unconscious mind wants you to know, or is there anything you're not getting which if you got it, would allow the problem to disappear?

14. Is there a purpose for this problem? Is there a reason for this problem? Ask your unconscious mind.

15. Is it OK with your Unconscious Mind to support us in permanently, positively removing this problem and for it to allow you to have an undeniable experience of it, when we are complete?

Mark Shepard, NLPT—Master Practitioner & Trainer of NLP, Hypnosis & Time Line Therapy™:
Rapid Results for Individual and Organizational Empowerment & Transformation
ItsNotJustAboutTheFood.com Copyright 2003, 2004, 2005, 2013, 2014 by Mark Shepard All Rights Reserved

Beliefs: Unconscious Filters of "Reality"

One way we can get leverage enough to change is to become aware of the unconscious beliefs that are operating constantly in the background like little computer software "add-ons"

The thing to remember is beliefs are not "true" but they get us certain results. Positive beliefs are no truer than negative or limiting beliefs they just get us more satisfactory results.

The other piece about beliefs that we need to get into is the fact that every limiting belief that is currently causing a problem has at it's core a positive intention.

Sometimes it's tricky to even elicit what the limiting belief is on your own which is why it is helpful to have a coach or someone else read the questions below and write them down. The best way to answer these is without thinking. Just blurt out what comes up IMMEDIATELY for you when you hear the questions.

1. If I get what I want then *I have to figure out other things to do*
   (what would you lose or could go wrong if you get what you want?)

2. Getting what I want would mean *that I would probably be more selfish. I will focus more on own needs*
   (What would it mean negatively about you or others if you got what you wanted?) *Not giving others what they want.*

3. *Fear*
   causes things to stay the way they are now. *(What prevents things from changing?)*

4. Getting what I want will make *other people feel bad*

   (What problems could be caused by getting what you want?)

5. The situation will never change because *I can't figure out why how else to spend my time.*

(What constraints or blacks keep things the way they are?)

6. It is not possible for me to get what I want because *I'm too emotional.*

(What makes it impossible for you to get what you want?)

7. I am not capable of getting what I want because *too emotional*

_____

(What personal deficiency prevents you from getting your outcome?)

8. This will never get better because *I don't know where I'll be accepted by the human race.*

(what will always prevent you from truly succeeding?)

9. I'll always have this problem because *I'm too insecure to move on.*

(What prevents you from reaching your outcome that can never be changed?)

10. It is wrong to want to be different because *people currently in my life want me to stay the same.*

(What makes it wrong or inappropriate to want to change?)

11. I don't' deserve to get what I want because *I do deserve it!*

_____

(What have you done, or not done, that makes you unworthy of getting what you want?)

Mark Shepard, NLPT—Master Practitioner & Trainer of NLP, Hypnosis & Time Line Therapy™:
Rapid Results for Individual and Organizational Empowerment & Transformation
ItsNotJustAboutTheFood.com Copyright 2003, 2004, 2005, 2013, 2014 by Mark Shepard All Rights Reserved

Chapter 9
Habits

Habits: Patterns of Thought & Behavior...

For many people their attempts to change negative patterns or habits in their lives and to replace them with positive ones, brings them right up against the wall of a seemingly un-cooperative unconscious mind.

Part of the problem is in the approach. We seem to think we can force change with our will power. One analogy of this is trying to lift your car by your own strength. Unless you are a professional weight lifter, it ain't gonna happen. And you can even hurt yourself trying. But get a simple tool like a jack, and even a child can raise the car.

> We are what we repeatedly do. Excellence, then, is not an act, but a habit.
>
> —Aristotle

We approach changing our habits, with our conscious minds when the very nature of a habit determines that it is in the realm of the unconscious mind. Think about it. When you were learning to drive a car. all the things you did at first were conscious weren't they?

> Any habit needs all its parts in order to function. If some parts are missing the habit is disassembled.
>
> —Carlos Casteneda

You had to literally be aware of things like. "Move foot from brake to gas." "Push a little on gas." "Push a little less." "Oh, look ahead!" "Turn steering wheel, oops! not so much!" etc...

Gradually, through practice, more and more of the work of driving got transferred to the realm of habit: your Unconscious Mind. So now, the act of driving is something that just happens in the background while you think about other things. So it stands to reason that in order to change a habit you have to actually approach it on the unconscious level as well as to take the necessary steps to install new habits.

> I have not come to health by wishing for it, laying myself in the hands of others, or ignoring the problems that were affecting it. I tried all of these approaches, of course, without success. I count my health today from the moments—when ill, dying or suffering physically—that I realized I had the wisdom within me for my healing. I count my health from the occasions when I took charge of my path to wellness. I count my health today from the times I looked kindly but unflinchingly at myself and began to change the habits that did not serve me.
>
> —Lenedra J. Carrol, The Architecture of All Abundance, p. 247.

Mark Shepard, NLPT—Master Practitioner & Trainer of NLP, Hypnosis & Time Line Therapy™:
Rapid Results for Individual and Organizational Empowerment & Transformation
ItsNotJustAboutTheFood.com Copyright 2003, 2004, 2005, 2013, 2014 by Mark Shepard All Rights Reserved

Habits: Patterns of Thought & Behavior (continued)

The other part of the problem is in the expectations we have. We think that eating a new way for a week will enable us to lose 100 pounds. or some magical diet pill or operation or personal trainer, or hypnotist will enable us to get what we want without having to take the time out from our busy schedule to actually do things differently for a long enough period of time for them to become installed as new habits. We want change without effort.

Now don't get me wrong, using hypnosis, NLP and Time Line will help to save time and will give you the leverage that a jack gives so that it becomes a lot easier and more possible to achieve your desired results. However, you still have to get out of your car, open the trunk, get the jack out, place it properly and start turning the crank.

I can teach you how to do this but ultimately you have to apply the principles consistently and persistently enough to lock in the new patterns...Blah, blah , blah!

Sorry, I didn't mean to get back on my "Response-Ability" soapbox. But it's crucial that you understand this. If you are overeating because you are stressed out from living a life where you are running around all day from before sunrise to after midnight doing, and doing and doing, you are not going to stop the overeating until you stop the larger pattern of "dis-ease" in your life.

> The word habit goes back to the Latin word meaning "what one has," and it developed into "habitus," which meant "how one is"- your personal state or condition. Etymologically, as well as practically, a habit is the recurrent outer pattern of a personal inner state. (using both word histories, "a habit" could be thought of as "an attitude" in motion)
>
> Your habits announce how you are, the ways of doing things you have put together that weave the fabric of your life…
>
> Your habits are metaphors for who you are.
> - Eric Booth, The Everyday Work of Art, p. 118

The next few pages contain exercises and other tools to help you to find out what it is you are doing now. Please use them fully. the first is a food log. For at least a week. Keep track of everything you put in your mouth and what is going on in your inner and outer world each time you eat. This will help to bring your eating habits into your conscious awareness.

The second or third week, keep track of your activities throughout the day. This is a powerful tool I use with my business clients as well. If you are doing too much make a note of the activities you do in a day that could be done better, or cheaper by someone else.

One of the stories I hear frequently (mostly from women but a few men as well) is that they are stressed and worn out doing all the home stuff, the laundry, the grocery shopping, the cooking and cleaning, as well as working in a high pressure jobs and they feel angry and resentful.

They eat the wrong foods because there was no time to do anything nice for themselves. They don't exercise because they have no time. But there are cleaning services, laundry services, live in nannies, etc. or they can choose to make other choices in their lives.

Sometimes work needs to be done in relationships so that each partner is carrying a fair share of the work.

Sometimes we simply need to let go of false expectations that a house must be perfectly neat or that we have to say yes to activities we don't want to do.

Mark Shepard, NLPT—Master Practitioner & Trainer of NLP, Hypnosis & Time Line Therapy™:
Rapid Results for Individual and Organizational Empowerment & Transformation
ItsNotJustAboutTheFood.com Copyright 2003, 2004, 2005, 2013, 2014 by Mark Shepard All Rights Reserved

Conscious Eating

1. **Stop! Rushing and gulping hurts the body.**

2. **Eat sitting down. Avoid eating in your moving car!**

3. **Bless the food to your use.** This doesn't have to be religious but involves imagining and visualizing this healthy food nourishing you and giving you energy.

4. **Focus on your meal.** Do nothing else while eating. No reading. No TV. Take small bites. Chew your food thoroughly. Explore moving the food from the front to the back of your tongue and from side to side to receive the most taste pleasure possible. Swallow completely before taking in the next bite. Savor the flavor. Enjoy the smell, taste, texture.

5. **Leave some food on your plate.**

6. **Notice how satisfied you feel. Focus on feelings of fullness and satiety.**

> In Clinical studies using Kirlian photography, an orange being eaten with attention and appreciation showed wave-like rays emanating from the fruit in all directions. One that was eaten quickly while the subject thought of events of the day showed minimal, dull activity. Dr. Leonard Laskow in his best-selling book, *Healing With Love* compellingly explores the idea that food consciously blessed before eating is measurably different than food that is not. He gives many examples of techniques for using the energy of love to Improve our health. Attention to color, beauty, and presentation in our meals has also been shown to add vitality to food.
> —Lenedra J. Carroll, The Architecture of All Abundance p. 243-244

Please Note: Take care of your nutrition needs throughout the day. This means making sure you keep healthy snacks and water with you. Cook or prepare enough healthy food ahead of time so you can easily heat up a nutritious meal even if you are tired or busy. Personally I would also make sure to support my body with proper herbal and vitamin supplements.

The point is to bring the act of putting food into your mouth into a positive, healthy consciousness.

"Hand to Mouth" Weight Reduction Log:

Please keep track of **everything** you put in your mouth for a full week. **Use a separate sheet(s) for each day.** Make a note of the context. Where were you? Who were you with? What were you thinking? What was your emotional state before and after each occasion? Feel free to make additional copies for yourself.

Time:	What?	Where?	Who?
Thoughts/State Before:		Thoughts/State After:	

Time:	What?	Where?	Who?
Thoughts/State Before:		Thoughts/State After:	

Time:	What?	Where?	Who?
Thoughts/State Before:		Thoughts/State After:	

Time:	What?	Where?	Who?
Thoughts/State Before:		Thoughts/State After:	

Time:	What?	Where?	Who?
Thoughts/State Before:		Thoughts/State After:	

Time:	What?	Where?	Who?
Thoughts/State Before:		Thoughts/State After:	

Time:	What?	Where?	Who?
Thoughts/State Before:		Thoughts/State After:	

Time:	What?	Where?	Who?
Thoughts/State Before:		Thoughts/State After:	

Mark Shepard, NLPT—Master Practitioner & Trainer of NLP, Hypnosis & Time Line Therapy™:
Rapid Results for Individual and Organizational Empowerment & Transformation
ItsNotJustAboutTheFood.com Copyright 2003, 2004, 2005, 2013, 2014 by Mark Shepard All Rights Reserved

Activity Log

What's your time worth? You can start with what you earn through your work. But what about the true value of your life? If you knew you were going to die tomorrow and could buy an additional day what would you be willing to pay? What would it be worth to spend a quiet (or not-so quiet) hour playing with your kids or grandkids? Please check out my song "Best Day Of Your Life"

Time	Activity	Pleasure scale (1-10)	Cost to Hire

Interrupting Your Old Patterns & Habits

In order to interrupt the old patterns we have to know what they are and how we do them.

Think about this: When you brush your teeth how do you do that? I mean, what do you do first? What do you do next? Do you wet your toothbrush? in hot or cold water? do you put a smidge of tooth paste on the brush or do you fill up all the bristles? Do you wet your toothbrush again or not? do you brush your top teeth or your bottom teeth first? How long do you brush for and when you are done do you rinse and tap the tooth brush on the side of the sink or just shake off the excess water?

However you do this, it is more than likely you do it the same way every time don't you? In NLP we call this a "Strategy" And you might be surprised to know that you have a strategy for virtually everything you do, from brushing your teeth to falling in love or out of love, to yes, knowing when it's time to feel anxious or fearful or confident or...that it's time to eat, or time to sit like a lump on the couch watching reruns of the shopping channel...

Normally, when I work with a client I will elicit his or her strategy for doing whatever problem they've come to me for help with. I can often pick up the strategy just from a client's eye patterns. It's a bit of a challenge for you to do this on your own because these strategies are usually unconscious.

However, by asking yourself the following series of questions you should be able to get a pretty clear idea of how you do whatever it is you have been doing that has resulted in the undesirable behaviors that brought you here. Or do this with a friend.

1. How do you know it's time to _____?
    (the undesirable behavior)

2. What's the very first thing you do? _____? Do you think something?, Feel Something? Say something to yourself? Get a picture of something?

    _____

3. What do you do next? Do you think something?, Feel Something? Say something to yourself? Get a picture of something?

    _____

Mark Shepard, NLPT—Master Practitioner & Trainer of NLP, Hypnosis & Time Line Therapy™:
Rapid Results for Individual and Organizational Empowerment & Transformation
ItsNotJustAboutTheFood.com Copyright 2003, 2004, 2005, 2013, 2014 by Mark Shepard All Rights Reserved

4. What next? _____

5. What Next? _____

6. What Next? _____

7. What Next? _____

8. What Next? _____.

Keep asking yourself until you get the whole strategy. For more help. Listen to my CD "Strategies: How to find out how you do the stuff that drives you crazy...so you can change it now!"

A really important question to ask yourself is: Have I ever "forgotten" to do this behavior? If you've ever forgotten to do the behavior, you want to explore what it was that caused you to forget to do the problem...eliciting the strategy for that is even more important than finding out how you do the problem.

The whole point of this is that once you know "how" you do something you can actually do things differently. The reality is that any habit is like a table. It needs all it's legs to stand. if you take one piece out of the puzzle of "problem" it can't stand. The strategy won't run.

Here's an example:

How do I know it's time to eat Ice Cream? This was my original strategy that I have long since replaced with a healthier one.

1. Well first I have to have a bit of a time break. It's usually after I've eaten something good like lunch or dinner and I start thinking about something for dessert...or sometimes I just want a little treat or pick me up in the middle of the day and I'll have some ice cream while I'm waiting for it to be time to do something else...If I'm really busy I will often forget about the ice cream. So I usually need a bit of a lull or some unstructured time.
2. Then, I get a picture of my refrigerator and I see the container of Starbucks Java Chip ice cream sitting there in the freezer...I imagine it's smooth texture and the pleasure I'll get from slowly melting it's rich coffee flavor in my mouth....
3. Then I get up go to the fridge, dish it up and eat it.

That's a very simple strategy. In order to interrupt it I first have to recognize it as a problem and decide to change it. What I would do then would be to see if I could scramble the strategy. I could keep the strategy from running merely by staying really busy (doing things I enjoy doing or working on some project). Or by not having Starbucks Java Chip in the refrigerator. I could also change the picture of the ice cream in my mind to make it have freezer burn or that gooey gummy stuff in it. I could also focus on a half eaten bowl that got left under the living room couch and kind of got dusty and moldy and just sticky and gooey...Or I could shrink down the internal picture I have of the Ice cream and move it down and to the left, which makes things less attractive for me.

This is often not the only intervention I will do but it is a good first step. Sometimes, it's enough in and of itself to help people change.

I was feeling a little sad the other day and by asking myself "How am I creating this emotion?" I was able to shift it.

Notice that the presupposition in that question led me back to "Cause". I didn't ask, "Why am I so sad?" I didn't ask, "Why is my girlfriend or the IRS or my next door neighbor so mean and heartless?" (or whatever).

I asked, "How am I creating this?" I am creating this. What is the process I am doing that is resulting in my current feelings of sadness.

The powerful question pulls me out of being a victim and gets me to take charge of my experience.

Give it a try!

Some other powerful questions that help to uncover your strategy for any particular behavior are:

"What do I have to focus on in order to have this problem or do this unwanted behavior?"

_____

_____

_____

"What do I have to ignore or pretend I don't know or what do I have to not notice in order to have this problem or do this unwanted behavior?"

_____

_____

_____

Submodalities:
Adjusting the Fine-Tuning on Your Internal Representations

Okay, let's assume you have a wee bit of a problem with ice cream... You've elicited your strategy and you know a lot about this pattern and how you run it time after time. One way to interrupt the pattern is to zero in on your internal representation of Ice cream itself.

For example: When I think of ice cream I have a picture. It's in color. It's right in the center and it's about where it would be on a table if I were sitting down and about to eat it. I am seeing it through my own eyes and I am anticipating the smooth and cold texture I will surely feel after I take a first bite. This is what I do by the way. What you do may be totally different. This is an example, only one of millions.

Now when I think of frozen yogurt or even of a kind of ice cream I don't care for (like maple walnut) I notice that the Yogurt or flavor I don't like is to my right and is a bit further out.

So now I know that by intentionally adjusting how I imagine ice-cream in my own mind, I can lower my desire for it. So now I take a moment and bring up the picture of Starbucks Java chip Ice cream and move it to my right and out a foot or so. Then I gently lock it in with an imaginary mental thumb tack or two.

Now I feel a lot less motivated to go and have another bowl... It's just a lot less in my face for one thing.

The next thing I can do is to literally take a picture of myself taking a walk or eating a piece of fruit or some other desired behavior and I can bring that to the center of my awareness, make it big and lock that in.

The strategy has been interrupted. So that when I think about ice cream I literally do something different than I had done previously.

I can now repeat this pattern to neurologically lock it in even deeper and give myself other behavioral options when I have a few minutes of free time after a meal or while I'm waiting for the next thing...

In order to help you do this for yourself I've provided the following check lists so you can easily check off what you are doing internally. You can also use the CD to guide you through this.

Mark Shepard, NLPT—Master Practitioner & Trainer of NLP, Hypnosis & Time Line Therapy™:
Rapid Results for Individual and Organizational Empowerment & Transformation
ItsNotJustAboutTheFood.com Copyright 2003, 2004, 2005, 2013, 2014 by Mark Shepard All Rights Reserved

Submodality Shift in a Nut Shell:

1. Think of a food you would rather not desire.

2. As you think of that food do you get a picture?

3. As you think of that picture go through the list of submodalities to find out what are the unique characteristics of this picture. Be sure to check in and notice if you have feelings or sounds associated with this or not. It's important to make a note of these as rapidly as possible. Just go through the check list.

4. Clear your mental screen

5. Think of a food that may be similar to the one you want to like less but that you dislike (ie. if target food is ice cream, elicit something similar like frozen yogurt that you may be easily able to avoid).

6. As you think of that less desirable food do you have a picture?

7. As you think of that picture rapidly go through the list of submodalities for Food #2 and **notice where the differences are.**

8. Clear your mental screen.

9. Now take food #1 and change the picture of it you hold internally to match that of food #2. For example if food #2 was in black and white while food #1 was in color. Change Food #1 to Black and White. If food #2 was far away and Food #1 was close, move Food #1 farther away.

10. Lock in the new characteristics of Food #1 with an imaginary Tupperware seal or super glue or duck tape or a lock or a bunch of rivets or pins or tacks or screws or nails etc.

Interestingly, since I originally wrote this section of the book back in 2005, I have literally stopped eating Starbucks Java Chip ice cream. I DID eat it one time when my mom got it for me when I visited her. I WAS able to eat it to be polite, but it did NOT re-trigger my addiction/compulsion/craving. Perhaps the very act of writing about this Submodality example, I had to actually do it internally… I do occasionally get ice cream but rarely have it in the house and when I do have it I enjoy the hell out of it without guilt or shame! But then I'm done with it for quite a while.

Ice cream no longer controls me! Same is true for chocolate chip cookies. This is such a simple process. Yet it is POWERFUL! PLAY WITH IT! Practice it. Enjoy!

Mark Shepard, NLPT—Master Practitioner & Trainer of NLP, Hypnosis & Time Line Therapy™:
Rapid Results for Individual and Organizational Empowerment & Transformation
ItsNotJustAboutTheFood.com Copyright 2003, 2004, 2005, 2013, 2014 by Mark Shepard All Rights Reserved

Submodality Checklist
Food #1: _____

Visual

[ ] B & W [ ] color

[ ] Bright [ ] Dim

Location: [ ] Near [ ] Far

[ ] life-size [ ] smaller [ ] Larger

[ ] **Associated?** (through your eyes)

[ ] **Dissociated?** (Looking as an observer)

[ ] Focused? [ ] Defocused?

Focus: [ ] Changing? [ ] Steady?

[ ] **Framed?** [ ] **Panoramic?**

[ ] **Movie?** [ ] **Still?**

Movie - [ ] Fast [ ] Normal [ ] Slow Motion?

Kinesthetic: any feelings important?

Location

Size

Shape

Intensity

Steady

Movement/Duration

Vibration

Pressure [ ] Soft [ ] hard

Weight [ ] Light [ ] Heavy

Auditory: Any sounds important?

Location

Direction

[ ] Internal? [ ] External?

[ ] Loud? [ ] Soft?

Tempo: [ ] Fast? [ ] Slow?

Submodality Checklist
Food #2: _____

Visual

[ ] B & W [ ] color

[ ] Bright [ ] Dim

Location: [ ] Near [ ] Far

[ ] life-size [ ] smaller [ ] Larger

[ ] **Associated?** (through your eyes)

[ ] **Dissociated?** (Looking as an observer)

[ ] Focused? [ ] Defocused?

Focus: [ ] Changing? [ ] Steady?

[ ] **Framed?** [ ] **Panoramic?**

[ ] **Movie?** [ ] **Still?**

Movie - [ ] Fast [ ] Normal [ ] Slow Motion?

Kinesthetic: any feelings important?

Location

Size

Shape

Intensity

Steady

Movement/Duration

Vibration

Pressure [ ] Soft [ ] hard

Weight [ ] Light [ ] Heavy

Auditory: Any sounds important?

Location

Direction

[ ] Internal? [ ] External?

[ ] Loud? [ ] Soft?

Tempo: [ ] Fast? [ ] Slow?

Swish Patterns

Computer Swish

1. Imagine the problem - <u>see it through your eyes</u>. notice the Visual, Auditory, Kinesthetic components or submodalities etc..

2. Imagine the ideal you - the you that would never have this problem. The ideal you - looking, acting, being - way beyond the problem. <u>See yourself in the picture</u>. tune this picture up. make it vibrant and bright if that makes it more compelling for you. You might want to make this a movie. Play with all the different ways to juice it up. Play a motivational sound track. (I love the national geographic special music)...

3. Imagine a computer screen - see the problem. Imagine the mouse in your hand. Notice the icon.

4. Click on the little X in the upper right hand corner and watch the problem disappear, revealing the new, desired state, the ideal you.

5. Repeat 7-21 times (If you repeat this enough times, the problem will have trouble returning).

6. Drag the problem to the trash folder - have it go to the same area where things are you would never do again. You can store it on an imaginary jump drive or external thumb drive and simply un plug it.

The Horizon Swish:

Take the old picture and push it all the way out to the Horizon just a little to the left of your vertical center line. push it all the wayout until it becomes a tiny speck and disappears.

Then bring in the new picture at a hundred miles an hour from that same point on the horizon. zoom it in big and bright and beautiful and compelling.

The Drop Down Zoom up Swish:

Take the old picture and fade it to black, down and to your left until it disappears Then zoom up the new picture from that spot. Remember to <u>see yourself</u> in the new picture. Also remember to tune up the positive sounds and feelings as well.

Anchoring Positive States

Introduction:

Pavlov's dogs. Or should we say Twitmeyer's Knees?

One day in the early 1900's a family doctor by the name of William Twitmeyer, was tapping a patient with that little hammer doctors use to test the knee reflex. Normal he would tap the knee and it would jerk a little bit. But this time Dr. Twitmeyer missed. He snapped the hammer back before it actually hit the knee. The knee still moved.

Twitmeyer excitedly wrote a paper about this and presented it to the AMA who as a group were basically not interested. Ivan Pavlov however, read the paper and continued to explore this phenomenon. Which we call the Pavlovian response. Pavlov showed his dogs a steak at the same time he rang a tuning fork. In a short time the dogs would salivate at the sound of the fork, even without a steak present.

Why are anchors useful for you?

We are being affected by stimulus response all the time. Every time you automatically stop at a red light or stop sign and then go when the light turns green. that is a visual anchor. Every time you hear a certain song and you suddenly remember exactly where you were the first time you heard it. Anchors are essentially presets in our body that enable us to respond without thinking. They can also be negative and disempowering so it's a good thing to know them about so that you can take charge of your own states by programming your own anchors, and learning how to cancel out any unhelpful anchors or triggers, isn't it?

What they are:
- Auditory: external and internal songs, sounds, voices, phrases. eg: I love you.
- Visual: external signs or symbols, internal pictures or movies.
- Kinesthetic: location specific triggers on your body that when touched activate specific feelings.

The Internal Representation

My Internal Representations determine my _____
and are made up of:

Visual:

The _____ that we hold in our mind.

Auditory:

The _____ that we hold in our mind

Kinesthetic:

The _____ that we hold in our mind

Auditory Digital (Self Talk)

The _____ that we hold in our mind

Mark Shepard, NLPT—Master Practitioner & Trainer of NLP, Hypnosis & Time Line Therapy™:
Rapid Results for Individual and Organizational Empowerment & Transformation
ItsNotJustAboutTheFood.com Copyright 2003, 2004, 2005, 2013, 2014 by Mark Shepard All Rights Reserved

Self Motivation

If I want to feel a certain way, all I have to do is to remember a time in the past when I felt that way. By bringing past memories into the present, I can be in charge of how I feel.

What's the best kind of memory to remember?

A good one or a bad one? **A good one!**

The difference between "Toward Motivation" and "Away From Motivation" is:

_____

_____

_____

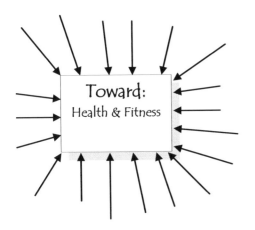

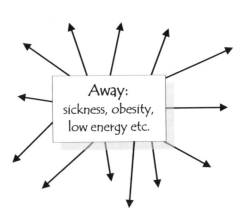

Away From Motivation produces _____ performance.

Toward Motivation produces _____ performance.

Mark Shepard, NLPT—Master Practitioner & Trainer of NLP, Hypnosis & Time Line Therapy™:
Rapid Results for Individual and Organizational Empowerment & Transformation
ItsNotJustAboutTheFood.com Copyright 2003, 2004, 2005, 2013, 2014 by Mark Shepard All Rights Reserved

Self Motivation

The top ten events in my life where I was totally motivated!

_____

_____

_____

_____

_____

_____

_____

_____

_____

_____

_____

_____

_____

_____

_____

_____

The Zoomer: Have the picture of Motivation come at you from across the room at 100 miles an hour and hit you and you're inside of it looking through your own eyes!

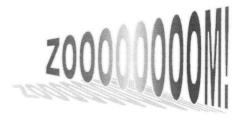

Mark Shepard, NLPT—Master Practitioner & Trainer of NLP, Hypnosis & Time Line Therapy™:
Rapid Results for Individual and Organizational Empowerment & Transformation
ItsNotJustAboutTheFood.com Copyright 2003, 2004, 2005, 2013, 2014 by Mark Shepard All Rights Reserved

The Resource Anchor

- Recall a time when you were totally motivated.
  Put it in your right hand.

- Recall a time when you were totally powerful.
  Put it in your right hand.

- Recall a time when you were totally loved.
  Put it in your right hand.

- Recall a time when you knew you could have
  whatever you wanted, a time when you knew you
  couldn't fail, when you could have it all.
  Put it in your right hand.

- Recall a time when you were totally energetic, full of
  energy.
  Put it in your right hand.

- Now open your right hand.
  Look at the shape...
  And the color...
  Feel how good it feels...
  and notice what it would say to you if it could
  talk....

- Now recall all those good things again.

- Recall a time when you were
  Totally powerful...
  Totally loved...
  Could have it all...
  Lots of energy, fired up...
  Put them all in your fist.

Here are some
additional desirable
states:

- Satisfied
- Secure
- Calm
- Assertive
- Courageous
- Fulfilled
- Appreciated
- Prosperous
- Healthy
- Fit
- Vigorous
- Attractive
- Beautiful
- Handsome
- Desired,
- Joyful

- Make your fist in a certain way and know that you can recall those feelings at any time, just make your fist that certain way.

- From now on when you have naturally occurring states of excellence, "stack" them on top of the ones you already have in your fist. The more you build this and tune it the more powerful a tool it is for when you need it most. You can also use other unique triggers, like a gentle pinch on your ear lobe or a certain song playing on your CD player or just in your head.

Mark Shepard, NLPT—Master Practitioner & Trainer of NLP, Hypnosis & Time Line Therapy™:
Rapid Results for Individual and Organizational Empowerment & Transformation
ItsNotJustAboutTheFood.com Copyright 2003, 2004, 2005, 2013, 2014 by Mark Shepard All Rights Reserved

94

State Vs. Goal

Anchoring is all about shifting states. Later on we'll explore setting goals and programming them into your future.

VALUE OR STATE	**GOAL OR OUTCOME**
Stated ambiguously	Stated specifically
Write "afformations"	Write goals/outcomes
You can have it now	Time is involved
No steps	Steps needed to get there (Get final step & work backwards)
Infinite	Measurable
Stated for self and/or others	Stated for self only

Q: Is "happiness" a goal or a state? _____.

Q: Is releasing 25 pounds a goal or a state? _____

Mark Shepard, NLPT—Master Practitioner & Trainer of NLP, Hypnosis & Time Line Therapy™:
Rapid Results for Individual and Organizational Empowerment & Transformation

Introducing Time Line Therapy®
a powerful tool for clearing the past
and programming the future.

In one of Master NLP Trainer Tad James's NLP courses, the students were doing an exercise where they broke up into small groups to practice various NLP techniques. One woman, associated into a traumatic event in her life. In other words she was suddenly "stuck" in a very uncomfortable memory where something "bad" happened. Because your unconscious mind doesn't recognize the difference between past, present and future, it was a traumatic as if it were happening "now".

Tad took her out in the hall to calm her down and it seemed like nothing in his NLP arsenal was working.

He asked her to float up above the event and observe it from a safe distance above. This usually helps but in this case it didn't. So intuitively, Tad asked her to float above the event and go farther back in time to at least 15 minutes before the event started and turn and observe the event from there...

Tad said it was almost as if someone had flipped a switch.

"It's gone!" she said.

Tad was very interested! "Are you sure?" he asked.

"Yes. Positive!" she replied.

Tad then had her go right down into the original traumatic event to make sure the emotions had disappeared. Even looking through her own eyes in that memory she felt neutral, clear and undisturbed.

From that original experience, Tad went on to develop Time Line Therapy as a model for permanent positive change. As a student of Tad and a certified master practitioner and master trainer of these techniques, it is my intention to give my clients and students an opportunity to get the benefit of Time Line Therapy™ techniques as a method of reinforcing the change work we've already done. Personally I use the CD with these techniques to clear any old Limiting Decisions that may come up in my own life.

This section is also good for people who can not locate a practitioner nearby. In the next section you will gain access to these tools and begin to use them for your own transformation.

Disclaimer: the author takes no responsibility for any experiences, positive or negative that the user may have as a result of using these techniques. Persons with severe psychological problems or trauma in their past are advised to do this work under the supervision of qualified professionals. For a list of these call my office or contact the Time Line Therapy Association.

What Are Beliefs and Limiting Decisions ?

"A belief is a generalization about a relationship between experiences."
- Robert Dilts

"Our beliefs are like unquestioned commands, telling us how things are, what's possible and what's impossible, what we can and can not do. They shape every action, every thought, and every feeling that we experience."
- Anthony Robbins, Awaken The Giant Within, p.24

"Things do not change; we change." - Henry David Thoreau

"If you can conceive it and believe it, you can achieve it!"
- W. Clement Stone, or Napoleon Hill, or Zig Ziglar (or all 3 of them!)

"If you have belief even as small as a mustard seed you can do amazing things, even move mountains."
- a well known Teacher from the suburbs of Jerusalem @ 30 AD

Beliefs address the world and how we operate in it. Beliefs guide us in perceiving and interpreting "reality".
- L. Michael Hall & Barbara P. Belnap, The Sourcebook of Magic:
A comprehensive Guide to NLP p.302

"Behaviors are organized around some very durable things called beliefs. A belief tends to be much more universal and categorical than an understanding. Existing beliefs can even prevent a person from considering new evidence or a new belief."
- Richard Bandler, Co-creator of NLP, 1982

Mark Shepard, NLPT—Master Practitioner & Trainer of NLP, Hypnosis & Time Line Therapy™:
Rapid Results for Individual and Organizational Empowerment & Transformation

Determining Limiting Decisions

In the "It's Not Just About The Food" Weight Loss Program, we use Time Line Therapy™ techniques to release negative emotions and limiting decisions. Generally, anything that is not a negative emotion such as Anger, Sadness, Fear, Guilt etc. is a Limiting Decision. There are also some additional clues for identifying a limiting decision. You'll know it's a limiting decision when it is described as:

1. **Anything you can't feel.** For example, "I don't feel happy"

2. **Negations:** As in the example above, anytime you hear a negation describing anything, which might be a Negative Emotion, you should be looking for a Limiting Decision. Examples include, "I'm not capable," I don't feel loved," and "I can't lose the weight I want."

3. **Comparatives:** Whenever you hear a comparison, such as "I wish I could lose weight," consider it a Limiting Decision. Comparatives include statements such as, "I have low self esteem," "I am not good enough," or "I want to feel better about myself."

4. **All beliefs:** What is not obvious is that any time we have a Limiting Belief we must have a Limiting decision which preceded it. Each time in the past when you adopted a Limiting Belief, a Limiting Decision preceded that acceptance. A limiting Decision precedes even the beliefs that were adopted from other people. If you find yourself saying "I don't believe I can do it", ask your self "When did I decide that?"

5. **Physiological Issues:** Many issues that result in physiological symptomology have their roots in decisions. (This includes all physiological symptoms that look like dis-ease)

6. **Accidents:** Many events in our past are the result of decisions that we made preceding the event. Even if this is not "true", when we accept our own creation of a past "accident" then we can un-choose the event and thus change our future.

7. **A Negative Emotion for which you are not "at Cause".** If there is a negative emotion for which you are not at cause, then it might be necessary to get the limiting decision for when you decided to create that negative emotion.
   (source: Tad James, Time Line Therapy ™   )

Belief Elicitation

_____: Fill in the blank with any attribute you desire: example: a slim, healthy body)

_____ is_____

People who have _____ are _____

People who don't have _____ are _____

People who have _____ have _____

People who don't have _____ have _____

People who have _____ get _____

People who don't have _____ get _____

Having _____ means you can _____

Having _____ means you can't _____

Without _____ I _____

With _____ I _____

With plenty of _____ I _____

With plenty of _____ I would have to stop _____

What people with plenty of _____ give up is _____

What people with plenty of _____ have to do to continue having plenty of _____ is

_____ -___

_____ causes _____

_____ creates _____

What is hard about _____ is _____

What is easy about _____ is _____

To have a lot of _____ one has to give up_____ _____

If I had more _____ I would _____

How I withhold _____ from myself is. _____

I can give myself _____ when I _____

Mark Shepard, NLPT—Master Practitioner & Trainer of NLP, Hypnosis & Time Line Therapy™:
Rapid Results for Individual and Organizational Empowerment & Transformation
ItsNotJustAboutTheFood.com Copyright 2003, 2004, 2005, 2013, 2014 by Mark Shepard All Rights Reserved

If I had more _____ I would have to give myself. _____

If I had more _____ I would allow myself. _____

If I had more _____ what would change is._____

If I had more _____ I would not permit._____

If I have more _____ people would._____

Living from a place of _____ is._____

What I "ought" to do to get more _____ is _____

History:

My mothers relationship with _____ was...
(how she received it, gave it, felt about it, talked about it)

My father's relationship to _____ was...

What I heard about _____ as a kid was...

"Misery and egocentricity
are synonymous.
To be miserable is to be the
center of the universe."

"There Is Nothing Wrong With You: Going beyond Self-Hate"
by Cheri Huber, Keep It Simple Books 1993

Got a good Excuse?

List all the reasons why you "Can't" make the changes in your life and body that you say you want to make.

_____

_____

_____

_____

_____

_____

_____

_____

_____

_____

Make a note of all the excuses which contain limiting decisions or beliefs.

Mark Shepard, NLPT—Master Practitioner & Trainer of NLP, Hypnosis & Time Line Therapy™:
Rapid Results for Individual and Organizational Empowerment & Transformation
ItsNotJustAboutTheFood.com Copyright 2003, 2004, 2005, 2013, 2014 by Mark Shepard All Rights Reserved

The Time Line

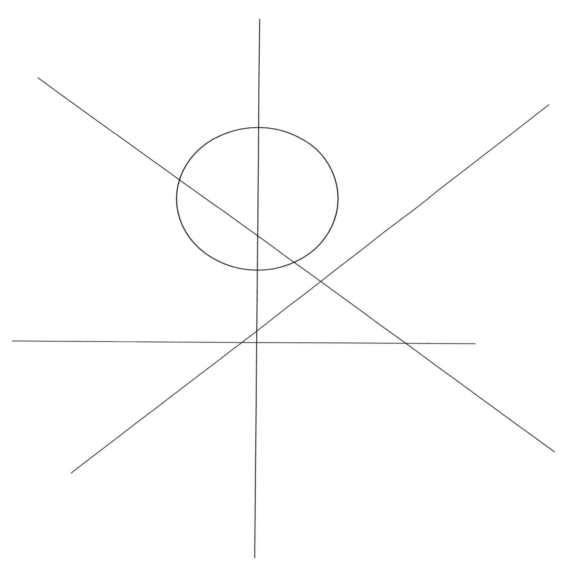

Where is your past?

Where is your future?

Mark Shepard, NLPT—Master Practitioner & Trainer of NLP, Hypnosis & Time Line Therapy™:
Rapid Results for Individual and Organizational Empowerment & Transformation
ItsNotJustAboutTheFood.com Copyright 2003, 2004, 2005, 2013, 2014 by Mark Shepard All Rights Reserved

Releasing Negative Emotions
and Decisions from the Past

#3. Float above line and at least 15 minutes before S.E.E. or moment of decision facing "now". Observe the event from before it happened. Now where are the emotions?

#2. Float up above the event as an observer. Preserve the learnings.

#1. Float above time line and float back facing significant emotional event

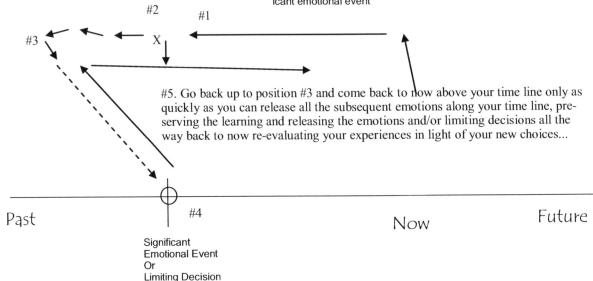

#5. Go back up to position #3 and come back to now above your time line only as quickly as you can release all the subsequent emotions along your time line, preserving the learning and releasing the emotions and/or limiting decisions all the way back to now re-evaluating your experiences in light of your new choices...

Past

Now

Future

Significant
Emotional Event
Or
Limiting Decision

#4. Once emotions have released, go right down into the event looking through your own eyes and check to make sure the emotions or decisions are gone.

Mark Shepard, NLPT—Master Practitioner & Trainer of NLP, Hypnosis & Time Line Therapy™:
Rapid Results for Individual and Organizational Empowerment & Transformation
ItsNotJustAboutTheFood.com Copyright 2003, 2004, 2005, 2013, 2014 by Mark Shepard All Rights Reserved

Chapter 10
Goals

Mark Shepard, NLPT—Master Practitioner & Trainer of NLP, Hypnosis & Time Line Therapy™:
Rapid Results for Individual and Organizational Empowerment & Transformation
ItsNotJustAboutTheFood.com Copyright 2003, 2004, 2005, 2013, 2014 by Mark Shepard All Rights Reserved

Program Your Future by Creating Memories For Your Future Timeline

1. **What do You Want? Be sure the goal is stated so it is S.M.A.R.T.**

2. **Get the last step:** "What is the last thing that has to happen so you know you got it?

3. **Make an Internal Representation:** Visual, Auditory, Kinesthetic, Olfactory, Gustatory

4. **Step into the Internal Representation and look through your own eyes** (associated).

5. **Adjust the SubModalities**—Adjust them for the most positive Kinesthetic or for the most "real" feeling.

6. **Step out of the Internal Representation**— Watch your self through the eyes of an observer (dissociated)

7. **Take the Internal Representation and Float above Now**.

8. **Energize the Internal Representation with four deep breaths:** Breathe in through the nose, out through the mouth and blow all the energy into the Internal Representation.

9. **Float out into the future:** Take the Internal Representation and float above the Time Line out into the future.

10. **Insert the Internal Representation into the Time Line:** Let go of the Internal Representation and let it float right down into the Time Line.

11. **Notice the Events between then and now re-evaluate themselves to support the goal.**

12. **Float back to now.**

Mark Shepard, NLPT—Master Practitioner & Trainer of NLP, Hypnosis & Time Line Therapy™:
Rapid Results for Individual and Organizational Empowerment & Transformation
ItsNotJustAboutTheFood.com Copyright 2003, 2004, 2005, 2013, 2014 by Mark Shepard All Rights Reserved

S.M.A.R.T. Goals

Goal: *"An aim or an end in mind"*
Aim relates to direction
End relates to outcome

Avoid the word "want".

Instead use:
- "I now have..." or
- "I now experience..."

S
Specific
Simple

M
Measurable
Meaningful to you

A
As if now
Achievable

R
Realistic
Responsible/Ecological

T
Timed
Toward What You Want

Mark Shepard, NLPT—Master Practitioner & Trainer of NLP, Hypnosis & Time Line Therapy™:
Rapid Results for Individual and Organizational Empowerment & Transformation
ItsNotJustAboutTheFood.com Copyright 2003, 2004, 2005, 2013, 2014 by Mark Shepard All Rights Reserved

For Example:

Not quite right:

I want to weigh _____ pounds by _____.

I don't want to be overweight any more.
I don't want to feel tired anymore.
I wish I could lose 100 pounds by next week...

Right:

It is _____. I now weigh _____.
           date   desired wt

I am currently wearing size _____.

I am feeling slim and trim, fit and full of energy , I maintain healthy habits of exercise, nutrition and rest daily.

Simple, **M**easurable, **A**s if now, **R**ealistic, **T**imed.

A typical example of results from using this process:
I recently had a client who came and did great work releasing and clearing huge chunks of negative emotional material. He went on to easily and effortlessly lose approximately 20 pounds.

He gave me a call a month or two after our last session and came in to do a reinforcement and goal setting session. He was going on a cruise with his wife and several friends and wanted to return a week later having lost an additional pound.

We set up the goal according to the "SMART" guidelines, inserting a proper picture of himself returning one pound lighter. Then he went off on his vacation. When he returned he was happy to say that he had indeed lost an additional pound while several of his friends had gained weight. One friend gained close to 15 pounds!

I saw him again for a reinforcement session just before the Christmas holidays. He had lost an additional 10 pounds and was now going to the gym 3 times a week with a buddy.

This process works.

Write Down What You Want

State vs. Goal

Value or State	Goal or Outcome
Stated Ambiguously	Stated Specifically
Write affirmations	Write goals/outcomes
You can have it now	Time is involved
No Steps	Steps needed to get there (get final step and work backwards)
Infinite	Measurable
State of Self and/or others	Stated for self only

Goals for Ten Years:

Goals for Six Years:

Goals for Three Years:

Goals For One Year:

Goals For Six Months:

Goals For One Month:

Mark Shepard, NLPT—Master Practitioner & Trainer of NLP, Hypnosis & Time Line Therapy™:
Rapid Results for Individual and Organizational Empowerment & Transformation
ItsNotJustAboutTheFood.com Copyright 2003, 2004, 2005, 2013, 2014 by Mark Shepard All Rights Reserved

How To CRUSH Anxiety
For more on this, visit www.CRUSHanxiety.com

Steps to relieve anxiety:

Float out above your time line towards the future and turn around and look back towards now 15 minutes after the successful completion of the event you thought you were anxious about....Ask yourself "Now where's the anxiety?"

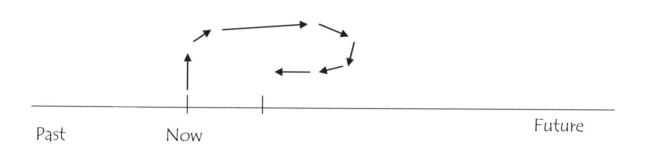

Past   Now   Future

Steps to programming your future: (making sure you goal is SMART)
1. Insert picture of you (seeing yourself in the picture) the way you want to look, feel, be etc. into your time line.
2. Then turn and look back towards now seeing all the steps needed to bring you to that desired goal.
3. Float back to now.

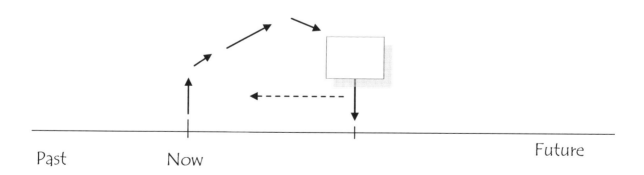

Past   Now   Future

Mark Shepard, NLPT—Master Practitioner & Trainer of NLP, Hypnosis & Time Line Therapy™:
Rapid Results for Individual and Organizational Empowerment & Transformation
ItsNotJustAboutTheFood.com Copyright 2003, 2004, 2005, 2013, 2014 by Mark Shepard All Rights Reserved

The Nature of the Universe

1. The Universe is made up of pure intelligence -It's basic nature is MIND.

2. Reality is not what I see. It is vibration—composed of frequencies.

3. Every thought or mental state has its own vibration. The universe will give you what you dwell upon.

4. The Universe demands balance—Everything has its opposite.

5. We are always compensated for what we do.

Mark Shepard, NLPT—Master Practitioner & Trainer of NLP, Hypnosis & Time Line Therapy™:
Rapid Results for Individual and Organizational Empowerment & Transformation
ItsNotJustAboutTheFood.com Copyright 2003, 2004, 2005, 2013, 2014 by Mark Shepard All Rights Reserved

Chapter 11
Reinforcement

Mark Shepard, NLPT—Master Practitioner & Trainer of NLP, Hypnosis & Time Line Therapy™:
Rapid Results for Individual and Organizational Empowerment & Transformation
ItsNotJustAboutTheFood.com Copyright 2003, 2004, 2005, 2013, 2014 by Mark Shepard All Rights Reserved

Reinforcement

When I first started doing this work as a practitioner I was very much into the idea that with NLP, Hypnosis & time line used together, change was so profoundly dramatic and long term that it eliminated the need to do a continual program of follow up work.

Then, in the process of training one of my associates, I got to be the Guinea pig. Up to this point, except for when I was in training myself, I hadn't had someone else to do the Time Line Therapy™ release work with me. I had been just doing it on my own. What happened changed my entire view of how to approach working with others.

I released huge chunks of material and I felt incredible. I felt like I was healed. done. Ready to move on to a better life. And then three days later, a related but different issue came up in my life...It was really intense and the following week I needed another session to address that piece.

The reality of the transformational process is that we are like an onion. Your unconscious mind has multiple layers of emotions, and beliefs that it may need to bring up and out to release, so there is a process here.

I also have to say that the most intense issues that I've released with Time Line have generally not recurred. Different aspects or contexts have come up following a release and needed to be addressed. But the main changes, stuck.

So in the process of releasing the negative emotions and limiting beliefs that are underlying your experience of your body, there may be a continual process of release and reinforcement for a while. This doesn't mean you are not doing it right, or that it doesn't work, it just means that you are in a process that takes some time. In fact that is one of the prime directives of the unconscious mind, that long term projects need repetition.

Looking back on the issues I was working on when I first started my healing journey almost 20 years ago, I can see how I am a completely different person. I can also see how every setback was just a blip in the road. At the time, I remember thinking, "Geez, I'm doing all this healing work, why don't I feel better?" With NLP and Time Line I definitely felt better and was more in charge of my experience than ever before, but, I wasn't "done".

We are never "done". That's why reinforcing the changes you've made is so vital. Practice changing your focus, using your physiology to shift out of a negative place. And, there may be another piece that has come up for release, so stop fighting that and address it.

The biggest challenge in this area with my weight loss clients is when they haven't lost weight every day. Over the course of a few weeks, they may gain a pound or two and they panic and get depressed and frustrated. The point is not to ask "why isn't this working" the point is to ask, "Is there something I am not addressing?"

Sometimes we don't' want to hear that. The reason drugs and surgery are so popular in this country is we want the quick, instant fix.

One of my clients was telling be about a co-worker of hers who "got the operation" and was looking great, lost a huge amount of weight. But she was still eating and thinking the same old way that got her fat in the first place..."

It is always my intention to assist people to get consistent, measurable, noticeable results in their lives whether we are working on weight loss, personal achievement, relationships, fears and phobias, habit control or whatever. Some issues can be dealt with quickly and easily and they never come back. Other issues need a long term approach that includes the willingness to look at every area of your life that may be contributing to the symptom we are addressing.

Essentially that is the meaning of a "Holistic" approach.

If you have made some changes working with me and notice that you aren't so full of anger any more or sadness or guilt, yet haven't started losing weight as quickly as you want, the next step is to look at your life. What are you holding on to that you need to let go of? What are you not dealing with? A number of people I've worked with, want to lower their stress without doing less in their lives! They want me to lower their stress so they can feel good as they continue to run around like maniacs taking their kids to a million places, cleaning the house, cooking the meals, shopping, going to PTA meetings, and working full time. You suggest to these people that they take some time for themselves and they just can't see how it's possible. It's like "how dare you suggest I change!". Or "How dare you suggest that I take care of my own needs first!". We have a lot of cultural programming to do for others first.

A classic example of this is given by Dr. Tad James. He worked with a man who needed to lose several hundred pounds. One of the things that had to change was the people he was hanging out with. They drank and smoked and were extremely negative. This client understood that he couldn't continue to do the same things that got him fat and expect to get thin. He began to make new friends and to go different places.

Change is possible when you say "no" to the old pattern. So maybe the underlying belief is that you don't have permission to say no and that shows up when someone hands you a big piece of gooey dessert. Or the reason you are reaching for the chips and pretzels before dinner is that you tried to do too much during the day and you didn't keep healthy snacks with you. Or perhaps there is still an emotional piece that hasn't been addressed to the satisfaction of your unconscious mind.

Mark Shepard, NLPT—Master Practitioner & Trainer of NLP, Hypnosis & Time Line Therapy™:
Rapid Results for Individual and Organizational Empowerment & Transformation
ItsNotJustAboutTheFood.com Copyright 2003, 2004, 2005, 2013, 2014 by Mark Shepard All Rights Reserved

The point is to stay with the process and with yourself. Treat yourself with the same love and compassion you would want from someone else...or that you would give to your cherished 4 year old child or niece or nephew.

Some times there are choices we make but we pretend that we don't have a choice. I don't mean to sound unsympathetic on this but...<u>we always have a choice</u>. Right now I could be on a beach in California instead of looking out my window into a sunny but cold March day in Albany NY. But I chose to be here with you. Stay with yourself. Keep reinforcing the good work you are doing. Be willing to accept that this is a journey with hills and valleys. You will get there. *You are getting there.* Imagine yourself there. Keep moving towards what you want. You are magnificent.

I have a number of clients who have worked with me for a couple of months and have not yet begun dropping the massive amounts of weight they thought they would, and yet they report back on amazing changes in many areas of their lives. In those cases there is almost always a great deal of underlying healing that is taking place. It's like the weight was the trigger that got them to seek help. If they made too much progress, too fast with that, they wouldn't be as likely to work on the root causes.

For me the motivating "problem with a purpose" was my seeming inability to get my music out into the world. After 5 years of intense work on myself I was finally making a living as a kid's musician. However, I wasn't satisfied because I still had hundreds of "Grown-up" songs that weren't being heard.

And my income was never steady or dependable. The fact that I didn't get "Exactly" what I wanted right away motivated me to continue to make changes in myself in order to resolve this. 10 or more years later, I was frustrated enough to keep searching until I found NLP.

I immediately began making dramatic changes in my life but even then, like the Jet Airliner that is off course 90% of the time, there were adjustments and course corrections, things I had to learn and integrate. Now 25 years after beginning this healing journey I'm truly beginning to fully integrate music into a much larger (and more satisfying) framework. If I had been successful right out of the box with music I might not have done the work... I remember complaining in the beginning, "if this is such great healing stuff why aren't I already rich and famous? I've been working on this for months!"

So the question to ask is not "Why isn't this working?" The question to ask your unconscious mind is:

"What is it I'm not getting, which when I get it, will enable me to lose the weight I want to lose and then permanently maintain the lean, high energy body I want, easily and sustainably?"

Mark Shepard, NLPT—Master Practitioner & Trainer of NLP, Hypnosis & Time Line Therapy™:
Rapid Results for Individual and Organizational Empowerment & Transformation
ItsNotJustAboutTheFood.com Copyright 2003, 2004, 2005, 2013, 2014 by Mark Shepard All Rights Reserved

Why is it possible?
The "Science" of Afformations

This is not technically "NLP" because I first began to use Afformations after reading a book by Noah St. John entitled, "Permission to Succeed". He coined the phrase "Aff**o**rmations" to distinguish them from "Aff**i**rmations". It is simply the use of positive empowering questions as a way to connect powerfully and directly to your unconscious mind. In essence an afformation is a fast form of self hypnosis.

You see, the brain tends to function like a computer. When we ask any question, your unconscious mind begins to look for supporting evidence and answers...It's the old garbage in, garbage out deal. Ask a crappy question and you get a crappy answer! Ask an empowering positive question get an empowering positive answer.

For a non empowering example: I was once assisting in the production of a national radio jingle. The producer was a lovely and wonderful man who was a delight to work with and who was probably making deep into the "six figures" income wise. There was some snag with the advertising agency or clients and I heard him whisper under his breath: "Why is it never easy?" I heard shortly thereafter that he left that business, depressed and frustrated. The point I'm trying to make is that we are already asking ourselves questions all the time. When we ask questions that presuppose or assume a negative answer, that is what we will get.

Here's a positive example: (please see the "Victory Song", "Arise, Arise", "Better Than Expected" , and "Field of Dreams" for songs that use this concept to reinforce positive questions):

An important piece of equipment began to show it's age by functioning erratically and showing signs of unreliability. I used it so much that I never had a chance to send it out for repairs. So I ordered a replacement by mail and requested UPS 2 day air so I would have the new amplifier in time for an important engagement. Well it did not come the day it was supposed to. Then the day of the gig, it started to snow like crazy. I had intended to use this amplifier instead of my full sound system at this event. Around lunch time it still had not arrived. I left the office to go home for lunch and sure enough the UPS delivery man came when I was gone. To my ultimate frustration he did not leave the delivery (even though I had specifically instructed that the package did not require a signature)

Meanwhile it started snowing like crazy and all of my equipment was in my trailer in the middle of a huge snow drift that was made bigger by the plow. I started to lose my usually calm demeanor. Because the presenters of the event refused to cancel (just because of a little snow) and because my amp hadn't arrived and because my old amp wasn't working reliably, I had to slog through the snow and haul out my full sound system. But of course in order to do that I had to remove all the seats from my mini van. It was just one of those situations where a person could get really stressed out...I caught myself starting to form an old habitual victim question on my lips..."Why does this always happen to me..." (sound of a LOUD buzzer here to interrupt the old pattern)

Once I caught myself beginning to ask that question I stopped and began to consciously say out loud:

Mark Shepard, NLPT—Master Practitioner & Trainer of NLP, Hypnosis & Time Line Therapy™:
Rapid Results for Individual and Organizational Empowerment & Transformation
ItsNotJustAboutTheFood.com Copyright 2003, 2004, 2005, 2013, 2014 by Mark Shepard All Rights Reserved

117

"Why does it work out better than I can possibly Imagine? WHY DOES IT WORK OUT BETTER THAN I CAN POSSIBLY IMAGINE? WHY DOES IT WORK OUT BETTER THAN I CAN POSSIBLY IMAGINE? WHY DOES IT WORK OUT BETTER THAN I CAN POSSIBLY IMAGINE?"

Practically chanting this afformation, I finished packing up the car and headed out into the snow...

After about 15 minutes of driving, the snow stopped! The sun came out! I got to the location nice and early and was met by a pleasant and courteous staff! The unloading was direct and easy, no stairs! And once I saw the room, a huge ballroom filled with tables for almost 200 diners, I saw at once that my new amplifier would never have been enough sound reinforcement for the entire room. If it had come on time, I would have shown up unprepared.

> Ever hear yourself saying "I'm sick and tired of _____"?
>
> One day I caught myself saying this and luckily noticed. I stopped.
>
> Now I say "Why am I healthy, energized and ready to **change this now?**"

It did certainly work out better than I could possibly imagine.

I could give you hundreds of examples of how this one affirmation has helped me and other people I've taught it to redirect our thoughts and transform life for the better.

Here are some others:

Why am I more and more healthy every day?
Why do I find myself eating only healthy nutritious foods?
Why do I find a way to touch the lives of others in a positive way?
How can I create the space in my life to consistently and healthfully exercise my body?
How can I take exquisite care of myself and my body today and everyday?
How can I use this information to powerfully and positively transform my life now?

Play time:
Your turn:

Why do you take a moment to come up with your own Afformations? How many "why" and/or "how" questions can you come up with?

_____

_____

_____

_____

_____

_____

(Afformations continued)

_____

_____

_____

_____

_____

_____

_____

_____

_____

_____

_____

_____

_____

_____

_____

_____

_____

_____

_____

_____

_____

_____

_____

_____

Reinforcement

Chapter 12
Values—
What's Important?

Mark Shepard, NLPT—Master Practitioner & Trainer of NLP, Hypnosis & Time Line Therapy™:
Rapid Results for Individual and Organizational Empowerment & Transformation

Could We Talk About Death For A Moment?

I don't mean to be morbid but we often forget that our bodies are the only thing separating us from the great beyond.

If you don't take care of your body, where will you live?

What is your life worth?

If you don't address the issues that are "killing" you, how long will you live? 1 year? 10 years? 20 years?

If you are more than 20 pounds overweight, you don't need me to tell you that it is a threat to your long term health. We all know that. We hear about it in the media all the time...

You have the tools to change your life in your hands. Use them. Keep using them. Use them even when you think it's all a bunch of baloney. These are the exact tools that top athletes use to pull themselves out of potentially defeating thoughts and behaviors, slumps and missed victories.

Choose to use your inevitable transition back into Spirit to motivate yourself to truly live in the wonderful body that takes you places and feels, sees, hears, smells, and tastes so much.

Check out the following song "This Could Be the Day that You Die" on the accompanying Thirsty For the Sky CD.

Keep in mind that it's just a reality check and a challenge to really start living your life now.

Mark Shepard, NLPT—Master Practitioner & Trainer of NLP, Hypnosis & Time Line Therapy™:
Rapid Results for Individual and Organizational Empowerment & Transformation
ItsNotJustAboutTheFood.com Copyright 2003, 2004, 2005, 2013, 2014 by Mark Shepard All Rights Reserved

The Very Best Day Of Your Life   **June 1997 edited 9/02**

You may sing like an angel, drive like Andretti,
March down the street in a shower of confetti
Consult with kings, donate money to the president
You might even brush your teeth with Pepsodent
But this could be the very day that you die (x2)

You could have plenty of insurance, stocks and bonds
Michael Jordan sneakers and a perfect lawn
You could have every single hair still on your head
You could be floating on air in your water bed
But this could be the very day that you die (X2)

Your time could run out before you even notice
You could leave in an elevator made by Otis
You could drop while you shop, while your drinking a soda
You might never come back from your trip to the Dakota
This could be the very day that you die (X2)

You could slip on a banana peel, drown in the tub
Get caught between a mother bear and her cub
Get run over by a fire truck
Have a heart attack in the middle of a good…book
This could be the very day that you die (X2)

This old guy I know says death is not the enemy
Death is our only worthy adversary
Death helps us focus on the stuff that really matters
One thought about death can cut right through the flatter-chatter
This could be the very day that you die (X2)

Now all that's been said and you're still not dead
You might want to start to live your life instead
You might want to do what you've left undone
You might want to learn to dance and play the drum!
This could be the very best day of your life (X2)

Mark Shepard, NLPT—Master Practitioner & Trainer of NLP, Hypnosis & Time Line Therapy™:
Rapid Results for Individual and Organizational Empowerment & Transformation
ItsNotJustAboutTheFood.com Copyright 2003, 2004, 2005, 2013, 2014 by Mark Shepard All Rights Reserved

The Jar—Getting Your Priorities Straight

When things in your life seem almost too much to handle, when 24 hours in a day are not enough, remember the mayonnaise jar...and the 2 cups of coffee...

A professor stood before his philosophy class and had some items in front of him. When the class began, wordlessly, he picked up a very large and empty mayonnaise jar and proceeded to fill it with GOLF BALLS. He then asked the students if the jar was full. They agreed that it was.

The professor then picked up a BOX OF PEBBLES and poured them into the jar. He shook the jar lightly. The pebbles rolled into the open areas between the golf balls. He then asked the students again if the jar was full.

They agreed it was.

The professor next picked up a BOX OF SAND and poured it into the jar. Of course, the sand filled up everything else. He asked once more if the jar was full.

The students responded with an unanimous "yes."

The professor then produced TWO CUPS OF COFFEE from under the table and poured the entire contents into the jar, effectively filling the empty space between the sand.

The students laughed.

"Now," said the professor, as the laughter subsided, " I want you to recognize that this jar represents your life. The golf balls are the important things: your Spirit, your family, your children, your health, your friends, and your favorite passions....things that if everything else was lost and only they remained, your life would still be full. The pebbles are the other things that matter like your job, your house, and your car. The sand is everything else-the small stuff. "If you put the sand into the jar first," he continued, "there is no room for the pebbles or the golf balls. The same goes for life. If you spend all your time and energy on the small stuff, you will never have room for the things that are important to you.

Pay attention to the things that are critical to your happiness. Play with your children. Nourish your relationships. Take care of your body. Play. Learn. Love.

There will always be time to clean the house and fix the disposal."

Take care of the golf balls first, the things that really matter. Set your priorities. The rest is just sand."

Mark Shepard, NLPT—Master Practitioner & Trainer of NLP, Hypnosis & Time Line Therapy™:
Rapid Results for Individual and Organizational Empowerment & Transformation
ItsNotJustAboutTheFood.com Copyright 2003, 2004, 2005, 2013, 2014 by Mark Shepard All Rights Reserved

One of the students raised her hand and inquired what the coffee represented. The professor smiled. "I'm glad you asked. It just goes to show you that no matter how full your life may seem, there's always room for a couple of cups of coffee with a friend."

Source: This is one of those forwarded e-mails you get from well meaning friends. Who knows where it originally came from. If you do, let me know and I'll give credit in future editions.

Mark Shepard, NLPT—Master Practitioner & Trainer of NLP, Hypnosis & Time Line Therapy™:
Rapid Results for Individual and Organizational Empowerment & Transformation
ItsNotJustAboutTheFood.com Copyright 2003, 2004, 2005, 2013, 2014 by Mark Shepard All Rights Reserved

Clarify Your Values

What's most important to you about your life?

What else? _____

What else? _____

What else? _____

What else? _____

What else? _____

What else? _____

What else? _____

What else? _____

What else? _____

What else? _____

What else? _____

What else? _____

What else? _____

What else? _____

What else? _____

What else? _____

What else? _____

What else? _____

What else? _____

What else? _____

Mark Shepard, NLPT—Master Practitioner & Trainer of NLP, Hypnosis & Time Line Therapy™:
Rapid Results for Individual and Organizational Empowerment & Transformation
ItsNotJustAboutTheFood.com Copyright 2003, 2004, 2005, 2013, 2014 by Mark Shepard All Rights Reserved

Values Hierarchy

Make a note whether these values are things you move towards or away from or some combination.

Prioritize your values: Towards| Away From

1. _____|_____

2. _____|_____

3. _____|_____

4. _____|_____

5. _____|_____

6. _____|_____

7. _____|_____

8. _____|_____

9. _____|_____

10. _____|_____

11. _____|_____

12. _____|_____

13. _____|_____

14. _____|_____

Is the way you life your life and the way you spend your time honestly consistent with your most important values? What steps can you take today to create a life that more truly reflects your values?

Mark Shepard, NLPT—Master Practitioner & Trainer of NLP, Hypnosis & Time Line Therapy™:
Rapid Results for Individual and Organizational Empowerment & Transformation
ItsNotJustAboutTheFood.com Copyright 2003, 2004, 2005, 2013, 2014 by Mark Shepard All Rights Reserved

What's important to you?

List the most important activities, and relationships in your life. How much time do you actually spend on them? Choose to make your reality reflect the value you place on these people and activities.

_____

_____

_____

_____

_____

_____

_____

_____

_____

_____

_____   _____

As far as all those activities that represent "sand". LIGHTEN UP ABOUT 'EM!

After all what's the use of a perfectly clean house and precisely folded laundry if you are not healthy or happy?

Mark Shepard, NLPT—Master Practitioner & Trainer of NLP, Hypnosis & Time Line Therapy™:
Rapid Results for Individual and Organizational Empowerment & Transformation
ItsNotJustAboutTheFood.com Copyright 2003, 2004, 2005, 2013, 2014 by Mark Shepard All Rights Reserved

Your Life's Purpose:

_____

_____

_____

_____

_____

_____

_____

_____

_____

_____

_____

_____

_____

_____

_____

_____

_____

Mark Shepard, NLPT—Master Practitioner & Trainer of NLP, Hypnosis & Time Line Therapy™:
Rapid Results for Individual and Organizational Empowerment & Transformation
ItsNotJustAboutTheFood.com Copyright 2003, 2004, 2005, 2013, 2014 by Mark Shepard All Rights Reserved

Chapter 13
Measure Your Progress

Mark Shepard, NLPT—Master Practitioner & Trainer of NLP, Hypnosis & Time Line Therapy™:
Rapid Results for Individual and Organizational Empowerment & Transformation
ItsNotJustAboutTheFood.com Copyright 2003, 2004, 2005, 2013, 2014 by Mark Shepard All Rights Reserved

Measure Your Progress

Hey. Your weight is not the only sign of progress is it? I can't tell you how many people get discouraged because they gained a half a pound in an otherwise excellent week. In that same week perhaps they began to exercise, changed their eating habits for the better, took the stairs instead of the elevator, parked their car on the other side of the Mall, and generally felt energized and good. Then they get on the scale and all the positive changes go out the window as they get really depressed about their "Failure." They first wail "What am I doing wrong?" (a negative Question that their unconscious mind tries to answer—see Afformations), then they delete all the positive things and make a picture in their brain of themselves getting fatter. Next, they pump a bunch of other toxic thoughts through their mind that set off a number of negative chemical reactions in the body.

The reality is that like the proverbial jet plane that is off course 90% of the time o n a flight from LA to Hawaii, (yet still arrives at it's destination), weight loss is a process. It's usually a process that takes months and sometimes years. It is a process that involves change at many different levels of your life. Some changes you make internally, others you make externally. The trick to staying on course is to make sure you focus on and notice all the areas of your life that are improving so that any one area doesn't cause you to abandon the course in over reaction to one piece of information that isn't to your liking.

So on the next pages I've created some aids at keeping track. If there are other things you can notice in your life that let you know you are making progress please add them.

How else can you acknowledge to yourself that you are making progress?

1. Typically we climb on the scale. (I suggest strongly that you avoid weighing yourself every day. Once a week is plenty. Once a month would be better but most people won't wait that long.)

2. Your body measurements. Measure yourself in every way you can think off when starting out. Then once a week or once a month do it again.

3. Percentage of body fat (you can have this checked out at a fitness center or even many modern scales can measure this)

4. Energy level. Use a 1-10 scale and keep track of it every day.

5. Altitude of your attitude. How's your happiness level? Use a scale of 1-10

as well.

6. Exercise: are you walking 3-5 times per week for 30-40 minutes? How many miles did you go? Keep a record and add it up at the end of each week. You can start with just 10 minutes a day!

7. Did you take the stairs today instead of the elevator? How many times?

8. Did you park your car as far out in the parking lot as possible? How many times?

9. Get a pedometer and keep a log of how many steps you've taken each week.

10. Did you do a Slow Burn exercise once a day?

11. Did you do the metabolism raising exercise at least once per day?

12. Did you visualize your ideal body at least once per day?

13. Did you write a page of Afformations?

14. Did you stop to count your blessings, smell the flowers, notice how beautiful the world is?

15. Look at the big picture. Add up all the ways you stayed on track this week. Give yourself a point for each action you took to take care of yourself.

Measure Your Progress

Other ways you can measure your progress:

- Did you do something kind for yourself today?
- Did you take time to breathe or a long relaxing bath or shower?
- Did you laugh?
- Did you make someone else laugh today?
- Did you notice someone in need who you could help in a positive way?
- Did you learn something today?
- Did you ask a loved one for help or assistance in a way that made you both feel good?

How else can you acknowledge to yourself that you are making progress?

1. _____
2. _____
3. _____
4. _____
5. _____
6. _____
7. _____
8. _____
9. _____
10._____

Mark Shepard, NLPT—Master Practitioner & Trainer of NLP, Hypnosis & Time Line Therapy™:
Rapid Results for Individual and Organizational Empowerment & Transformation
ItsNotJustAboutTheFood.com Copyright 2003, 2004, 2005, 2013, 2014 by Mark Shepard All Rights Reserved

Measure Your Progress

Make as many photocopies of this chart as you need.

Add a point for every positive action you took. eg. 1 point for every 10 minutes of walking. 1 point for every serving of green vegetables. 1 point for every glass of water you drank. 1 point for every time you stopped and counted your blessings or wrote a page of "afformations". 1 point for every meal you ate Consciously. You can even give yourself a point for each day you kept this log. Use the blank places for your own personal objectives.

	Mon	Tues	Wed	Thurs	Friday	Sat	Sun	Total: Points:
Walking								
Other Exercise								
Veggies								
Water								
"Afforma-tions" or Blessings								
Mindful Eating								
Energy (1-10)								
Attitude (1-10)								
Stairs & Parking								
Visualize Body								
Metabo-lism, set point etc.								
Self hyp-nosis CD								
Anchors								
Swishes								
Totals:								

Measure Your Progress

Your weekly check in.

	Weight	Waist	Arms	Thighs	Neck			Next set point?
Week #1								
Week #2								
Week #3								
Week #4								
Week #5								
Week #6								
Week #7								
Week #8								
Week #9								
Week #10								
Week #11								
Week #12								
Week #13								
Week #14								
Week #15								
Week #16								

Mark Shepard, NLPT—Master Practitioner & Trainer of NLP, Hypnosis & Time Line Therapy™:
Rapid Results for Individual and Organizational Empowerment & Transformation
ItsNotJustAboutTheFood.com Copyright 2003, 2004, 2005, 2013, 2014 by Mark Shepard All Rights Reserved

SHEPARD'S LAWS

(This is my answer to the famously defeatist body of thought called "Murphy's Laws", which I won't even bother to reprint here because in my opinion they should be treated like toxic poison for the mind...)

1. Why is it easier than it looks?

2. Why doe it usually take less time than you thought

3. Why is it that when things take more time than you thought they should but you look back on it with a curious mind, you will find there was a good reason for the delay and the delay actually served you in more ways than you might imagine.

4. Anything that can go right will go right. Anything that seems to be wrong is actually right, you just haven't gotten enough distance on it to see that clearly yet.

5. If you are open to the possibility that everything will work out better than you can possibly imagine, you begin to notice the many small things that are positive and in your favor. Corollary: if there is a best time for something to go right, it will happen at an even better time, even if it doesn't appear to be a better time at the time. If it seemed like it happened at the "wrong" time, get up above it in your mind and be open to the possibility that it only seems "wrong"...

6. If you perceive that there are four possible ways in which a procedure can go right, and stay open, then a fifth way, or even more ways to succeed, will promptly develop.

7. Left to themselves, things tend to change in one way or another or stay the same. Resisting change is evidence of a lack of creative thinking.

8. If you perceive that something cannot go right, look again, there is some way on some level that it is working out better than you can possibly imagine... If everything seems to be going wrong, you have obviously overlooked something.

9. Whenever you buy something you will see it somewhere else for a higher price.

10. Nature always sides with the hidden strength.

11. Mother nature is impartial.

Mark Shepard, NLPT—Master Practitioner & Trainer of NLP, Hypnosis & Time Line Therapy™:
Rapid Results for Individual and Organizational Empowerment & Transformation
ItsNotJustAboutTheFood.com Copyright 2003, 2004, 2005, 2013, 2014 by Mark Shepard All Rights Reserved

12. It is impossible to fail because there is no failure, only feedback.

13. Whenever you set out to do something, something must be done first, then second, then third and so on. The question to ask oneself is "How can I respond to this challenge in the most effective and appropriate way?"

14. There are no problems, only challenges, adventures, and opportunities.

15. If something seems like a problem, it is only a test and an opportunity to learn.

Shepard was a pessimist…

Thoughts?

_____

_____

_____

_____

_____

_____

_____

_____

_____

_____

_____

_____

_____

_____

_____

Five principles For Success

1.   Know your outcome.

2.   Take action.

3.   Have sensory acuity.

4.   Have behavioral flexibility.

5.   Operate from a physiology and psychology of excellence.

Mark Shepard, NLPT—Master Practitioner & Trainer of NLP, Hypnosis & Time Line Therapy™:
Rapid Results for Individual and Organizational Empowerment & Transformation
ItsNotJustAboutTheFood.com Copyright 2003, 2004, 2005, 2013, 2014 by Mark Shepard All Rights Reserved

Books:

NLP, Hypnosis and Time Line Therapy

Magic of NLP Demystified, by Byron Lewis & Frank Pucelik, Metamorphus Press, Portland OR, 1990, ISBN 1-55552-017-0

Changing Belief systems with NLP by Robert Dilts, Meta Publications, Capitoloa, CA, 1990 ISBN 0-916990-24-9

Time For a Change by Richard Bandler, Meta Publications, Capitola, CA, 1993 ISBN 0-916990-28-1

Structure of Magic I & II by John Grinder and Richard Bandler, Science & Behavior Books, Palo Alto, CA ISBN 08314-0044-7 and 08314-0049-8

Don't Shoot The Dog! The New Art of Teaching And Training by Karen Pryor, Bantam Books, 1984, 1999 ISBN 0-553-38039-7

Time Line Therapy & the Basis of Personality by Tad James & Wyatt Woodsmall, 1988 Meta Publications, Capitola, CA, 1990 ISBN 0-916990-21-4

Unlimited Power by Anthony Robbins, Simon & Schuster, NY 1986 ISBN 0-671-6008-0

Awaken the Giant Within By Anthony Robbins, Simon & Schuster, NY 1992 ISBN 0-671-72734-6

Permission to Succeed by Noah St. John, Health Communications, Inc. Deerfield Beach, FL ISBN 1-55874-719-2

Weight Loss, Nutrition, Fitness

The Neuropsychology or Weight Control by Steven A. DeVore, Dennis W. Remington, MD, A. Garth Fisher, PhD, Edward A. Parent, PhD., SyberVision Systems, Inc.

The Fat Fallacy by Will Clower, PhD, Three Rivers Press, NY 2002

Healthy Fats For Life by Lorna R. Vanderhaeghe & Karlene Karst, published by John Wiley and Sons Canada, Ltd. 2004

Grain Brain: The Surprising Truth About Wehat, Carbs, and Sugar—Your Brain's Silent Killers by David Perlmutter, MD, Little, Brown and Company, NY 2013

The Slow Burn Fitness Revolution by Fredrick Hahn, Michael R, Eades and Mary Dan Eades, Broadway Books (A Division of Random House) NY 2003

Virgin Coconut Oil—How it Has Changed People's Lives and How It Can Change Yours! by Brian and Marianita Jader Shilhavy, Tropical Traditions, 2004

- The Field: The Quest for the Secret Force of the Universe by Lynn McTaggart (www.thefieldonline.com)If there was any one book we would have to recommend in order to understand more fully the concepts in 'What the BLEEP,' it would have to be this best-seller. It may forever change your world view (if it hasn't changed already!). This examination of the Zero Point Field creates a picture of an interconnected universe and a new scientific theory, which makes sense of 'supernatural' phenomena.

- Molecules of Emotion: The Science Behind Mind-Body Medicine by Candace B. Pert A groundbreaking book that provides decisive and startling answers as to how our thoughts and emotions affect our health and our lives.

- Why God Won't Go Away: Brain Science and the Biology of Belief by Eugene G. D'Aquilli, Vince Rause, and Andrew Newberg, M.D. This engaging work examines the activity of the brain when God is experienced. Unique and thought-provoking.

- The Tao of Physics by Fritjof Capra One of the first books to explore the parallels between modern physics and Eastern mysticism. The Tao of Physics is a classic!

- The God Particle: If the Universe is the Answer, What is the Question? by Leon Lederman With humor and a passion for the unknown, Lederman takes you on a journey to discover the ultimate building blocks of matter to discover the illusive, primordial God Particle.

- The Power of Now: A Guide to Spiritual Enlightenment by Eckhart Tolle With simplicity and grace, Tolle reminds us to free ourselves from the dominance of our minds and liberates us from both past and future.

- A Hole in the Universe: How Scientists Peered Over the Edge of Emptiness and Found Everything by K.C. Cole Ms. Cole plunges into the void with today's top scientists and theorists, showing how the continuing search for the ultimate nothingness is leading to a profound new understanding of the origins and nature of the ever-changing Universe.

- Beyond Einstein: The Cosmic Quest for the Theory of the Universe by Michio Kaku Beyond Einstein takes readers on an exciting excursion into the discoveries that have led scientists to the brightest new prospect in theoretical physics today -- superstring theory. Co-authored by one of the leading pioneers in superstrings, Michio Kaku, and completely revised and updated with the newest groundbreaking research, the book approaches scientific questions with the excitement of a detective story, offering a fascinating look at the new science that may make the impossible possible.

- The Self-Aware Universe: How Consciousness Creates the Material Worldby Maggie Goswami, Richard E. Reed, Amit Goswami and Fred Alan Wolf This book proposes a new paradigm – a unifying worldview that integrates mind and spirit into science, embracing the development of a science that embraces all religions. At the core of the new paradigm is the centerpiece of consciousness as the Ground of all Being.

- The Science of Mind by Ernest Holmes The Science of the Mind was originally published in 1926 by the founder of the worldwide Religious Science movement. It is a true classic of spiritual literature, which clearly delineates how the mind effects one's life, and how by the useful application of that knowledge one's life becomes transformed.

- The Thunder of Silence by Joel S. Goldsmith This is a classic written by the internationally known mystic who brought clarity and understanding to the purpose and function of the mind. Mysticism and science merge in this masterpiece to bring greater awareness of the erroneous belief in duality which separates us from the realization of our Oneness with all being. It further presents the spiritual laws which enable us to live a life of peace, love and freedom, thus becoming instruments of divine expression

Testimonials:

Mark,

Words can never express how grateful I am for the time I have spent with you. When I first saw your name in the local Yellow Pages I instantly knew I had to find out more about your services and was somehow fortunate enough to bring you into my life. You patiently worked with me and helped guide me to a path of lifelong success.

I was then blessed again to be able to spend extensive time working with you when I was selected for the 8-Week Weight Loss Challenge. I can never repay you for the life lessons you taught me from June through July'04. My weight dropped by 20 lbs. in that time period and I lost numerous inches but the biggest change was to my mind, my thoughts have never been the same since!!

The concepts of Hypnosis, TimeLine Therapy, NLP , Swish Patterns and many more formerly foreign sounding phrases now mean a lot to me. I am able to use the principals and concepts you taught me to better all aspects of my life, not just my weight. I am constantly reminded of the priceless information you presented to me and it continues to make a difference in my daily life. You taught me that I am in control, only I can make change happen. Every day old behaviors feel more and more uncomfortable and the new habits seem more natural.

Even after the next few months of ongoing support are past I hope to be able to continue to work with you and learn from you. You are an amazing support in my life and your words stay with me even when I am not in your presence.

Thank you for everything.

Sandy Sarno

Made in the USA
Charleston, SC
18 March 2014